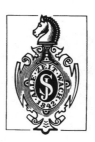

B. J. Cremin P. Beighton

Bone Dysplasias of Infancy

A Radiological Atlas

Foreword from R. O. Murray

With 55 Figures (124 Separate Illustrations)

Springer-Verlag
Berlin Heidelberg New York 1978

Professor Bryan J. Cremin, F.R.A.C.R., F.R.C.R
Head, Department of Radiology,
Groote Schuur and Red Cross Childrens Hospital,
University of Cape Town,
Rondebosch 7700, South Africa

Professor Peter Beighton, M.D., Ph.D., F.R.C.P., D.C.H.
Department of Human Genetics,
Groote Schuur Hospital,
University of Cape Town,
Observatory 7925, South Africa

ISBN-13: 978-3-642-48309-7   e-ISBN-13: 978-3-642-48307-3
DOI: 10.1007/978-3-642-48307-3

Library of Congress Cataloging in Publication Data. Cremin, Bryan Joseph. Bone dysplasias of infancy. Bibliography: p. Includes index. 1. Bones—Diseases—Atlases. 2. Bones—Abnormalities—Atlases. 3. Bones—Radiography—Atlases. 4. Infants—Diseases—Atlases. 5. Pediatric radiography—Atlases. I. Beighton, Peter, joint author. II. Title. RJ482.B65C73   617.3   78-17435

This work is subjected to copyright. All rights are reserved, whether the whole or part of the material is concerned specifically those of translation, reprinting, re-use of illustrations, broadcasting, reproduction by photocopying machine or similar means, and storage in data banks. Under §54 of the German Copyright Law where copies are made for other than private use, a fee is payable to the publisher, the amount of the fee to be determined by agreement with the publisher.

The use of registered names, trademarks, etc. in this publication does not imply, even in the absence of a specific statement, that such names are exempt from the relevant protective laws and regulations and therefore fee for general use.

© by Springer-Verlag Berlin Heidelberg 1978
Softcover reprint of the hardcover 1st edition 1978

Foreword

The tremendous expansion of medical knowledge during the last few decades, together with the introduction of many new diagnostic techniques, has demanded such a degree of specialisation that no single individual can be conversant with all the information available. More and more emphasis, therefore, has been placed on the importance of teamwork and close collaboration between associated disciplines. The bone dysplasias of infancy represent a classical example of this concept. Only a few years ago these heritable conditions were divided into a relatively small number of entities, for many of which "atypical variants" were accepted. More recent studies have resulted in appreciation and early recognition of a large number of these disorders, thanks to co-operation between paediatricians, radiologists, geneticists and biochemists. Not only may a reasonably accurate prognosis be offered for the affected child in many instances, but, almost of greater value, genetic counselling concerning the chance of subsequent offspring being similarly affected has become available to parents.

Most radiologists have little opportunity of becoming familiar with this rapidly widening field of diagnosis, so that the occasional case which may be encountered is likely to engender diagnostic difficulty. This Atlas should facilitate greatly the solution of the problem. It has been prepared by Professor CREMIN, an outstanding paediatric radiologist whose work has been known and admired by me for many years, in close collaboration with his colleague Professor BEIGHTON, a geneticist of great distinction. The combination of systematic assessment of the radiological evidence and the genetic characteristics of the conditions described provides a comprehensive account of the present state of knowledge. As the authors point out the field, as yet, has not been explored completely and the hope may be expressed that further information, when it become available, will be incorporated in future editions. The authors are to be congratulated on this excellent and up-to-date contribution to the literature of a difficult subject.

London, June, 1978   R. O. MURRAY

Acknowledgements

We are grateful to Dr. F. N. Silverman and Prof. J. W. Spranger for their opinion on cases that we have sent to them and to Dr. P. E. S. Palmer for reading and advising on the manuscript. We are greatly indebted to Mrs. Thelma Hochschild, Principal Radiographer at the Red Cross Children's Hospital for her untiring work in preparing the radiographs and for her assistance in correlating and arranging the material. We would also like to thank our departmental colleagues Drs. R. M. Fisher and M. Nelson. We are also indebted to Mrs. S. Henderson for her photography, to Miss B. Neumann, Mrs. G. Beighton, Mrs. B. Breytenbach and Mrs. J. Groom for typing the manuscript. We acknowledge the permission received from Drs. Toland, Perri, and Harris for Figures 5-3, 10-1 and 12-1 and to the Director of the Institute of Anthropology, Mexico City, for permission to use the illustration on the cover.

The authors acknowledge the following Journals for permission to use reproductions from their own publications; The British Journal of Radiology for Figures 3-2 (b, c), 4-2 (a), 5-1 (a, b, c, d), 6-1 (d, e), 8-4, 9-1, 10-4 (a, b); The Australasian Journal of Radiology for 11-2 (a, b, c), Radiology for Figure 2-3 (a, b) and Radiology for 2-3 (a, b).

We thank the South African Medical Research Council and the University of Cape Town Staff Research Fund for their financial support for our investigations.

Cape Town, June, 1978

Bryan J. Cremin
Peter Beighton

Table of Contents

Foreword   V

Acknowledgements   VII

Glossary of Useful Terms   XI

Comments on Terminology   XIII

Introduction   1

1. Clinical and Genetic Evaluation of the Neonate with Skeletal Dysplasia   3
2. Radiographic Techniques   9
3. Achondrogenesis   17
4. Thanatophoric Dysplasia   21
5. Asphyxiating Thoracic Dysplasia   27
6. Chondroectodermal Dysplasia   33
7. Lethal Short Rib-Polydactyly Syndromes   37
8. Chondrodysplasia Punctata   45
9. Campomelic Dysplasia   53
10. Achondroplasia   55
11. Diastrophic Dysplasia   61
12. Metatropic Dysplasia   67
13. Spondyloepiphyseal Dysplasia Congenita   71
14. Mesomelic Dysplasia   73
15. Larsen Syndrome   79
16. Cleido-Cranial Dysplasia   83
17. Osteogenesis Imperfecta Congenita   91
18. Hypophosphatasia   97
19. Osteopetrosis and other Sclerosing Bone Dysplasias   101

Appendix   108
Subject Index   109

Glossary of Useful Terms

Acromelia	Shortening of distal portion of limb
Acromesomelia	Shortening of the middle and distal portion of the limb
Appendicular	Dependent portions of the skeleton
Axial	Trunk portion of the skeleton
Campomelia	Bent limb
Clinodactyly	Deviation of a finger
Congenital abnormality	An abnormality which is present at birth, but not necessarily genetic
Diaphysis	Middle portion of the shaft of a long bone
Diastrophic	Twisted
Dysostosis	A defect in ossification or modeling
Dysplasia	Intrinsic growth disturbance
Dystrophy	Growth disturbance influenced by external factors
Hexadactyly	Six digits
Hypertelorism	Wide gap between the orbits
Mesomelia	Shortening of the middle portion of limb
Metaphysis	Extremity of the shaft of a long bone
Metatropic	Changeable
Micrognathia	Small jaw
Micromelia	Short limb
Nanism	Small stature or dwarfism
Phenotype	Outward expression of genetic constitution
Platyspondyly	Flattening of vertebrae
Polydactyly	Supernumerary digits
Post-axial	Ulnar or fibular side
Pre-axial	Radial or tibial side
Rhizomelic	Proximal portion of a limb
Siblings	Offspring of the same parent
Symphalagism	End to end fusion of contiguous phalanges
Syndactyly	Soft tissue or bony union between adjacent digits
Thanatophoric	Death bearing

Important terms used in clinical genetics are explained in Chapter Two.

Comments on Terminology

Because of the confusion in terminology concerning the bone dysplasias, a sub-committee of the European Society of Pediatric Radiology met in Paris in 1969 and elaborated a nomenclature that divided the Constitutional (Intrinsic) diseases of bone into those with unknown and known pathogenesis. The unknown group were further divided into osteochondrodysplasias (abnormalities of cartilage and/or bone growth and development), dysostoses (malformation of individual bones, single or in combination), and other groups.

The osteochondrodysplasias were subdivided into three groups, the first of which were defects of growth of tubular bones and/or spine that manifested (A) at birth and (B) in later life.

This portion of the nomenclature is given below:

Constitutional Diseases of Bones with Unknown Pathogenesis.

Osteochondrodysplasias (abnormalities of cartilage and/or bone growth and development)

1. Defects of growth of tubular bones and/or spine.

A) Manifested at birth

1. Achondrogenesis
2. Thanatophoric dwarfism
3. Achondroplasia
4. Chondrodysplasia punctata (formerly stippled epiphyses) (several forms)
5. Metatropic dwarfism
6. Diastrophic dwarfism
7. Chondro-ectodermal dysplasia (ELLIS-VAN CREVELD)
8. Asphyxiating thoracic dysplasia (JEUNE)
9. Spondylo-epiphyseal dysplasia congenita
10. Mesomelic dwarfism: type NIEVERGELT; type LANGER
11. Cleido-cranial dysplasia (formerly cleido-cranial dysostosis).

B) Manifested in later life

1. Hypochondroplasia
2. Dyschondosteosis
3. Metaphyseal chondro-dysplasia type JANSEN

4. Metaphyseal chondro-dysplasia type SCHMID
   5. Metaphyseal chondro-dysplasia type MCKUSICK
      (formerly cartilage-hair hypoplasia)
   6. Metaphyseal chondro-dysplasia with malabsorption and neutropenia
   7. Metaphyseal chondro-dysplasia with thymolymphopenia
   8. Spondylo-metaphyseal dysplasia (KOZLOWSKI)
   9. Multiple epiphyseal dysplasia (several forms)
  10. Hereditary arthro-opthalmopathy
  11. Pseudo-achondroplasic dysplasia
      (formerly spondylo-epiphyseal pseudo-achondroplasic dysplasia)
  12. Spondylo-epiphyseal dysplasia tarda
  13. Acrodysplasia
      a) Rhino-trico-phalangeal syndrome (GIEDION)
      b) Epiphyseal (THIEMANN)
      c) Epiphyso-metaphyseal (BRAILSFORD)

The nomenclature was revised in Paris at a further meeting in 1977 and the proposed first portion is given below:

1. Defects of growth of tubular bones and/or spine.

A) Identifiable at birth

   1. Achondrogenesis type I (PARENTI-FRACCARO)
   2. Achondrogenesis type II (LANGER-SALDINO)
   3. Thanatophoric dysplasia
   4. Thanatophoric dysplasia with Clover-leaf Skull
   5. Short rib-polydactyly syndrome type I (SALDINO-NOONAN)
      (perhaps several forms)
   6. Short rib-polydactyly syndrome type II (MAJEWSKI)
   7. Chondrodystrophia punctata
      a) Rhizomelic type
      b) Dominant type
      c) Other types
      d) Exclude symptomatic stippling in other disorders
         (ZELLWEGER syndrome, Warfarin embryopathy and others)
   8. Campomelic dysplasia
   9. Other dysplasias with congenital bowing of long bones
  10. Achondroplasia
  11. Diastrophic dysplasia
  12. Metatropic dysplasia (several forms)
  13. Chondro-ectodermal dysplasia (ELLIS-VAN CREVELD)
  14. Asphyxiating thoracic dysplasia (JEUNE)
  15. Spondylo-epiphyseal dysplasia congenita (SPRANGER-WIEDEMANN)
  16. Other spondylo-epiphyseal dysplasias recognizable at birth
  17. KNIEST dysplasia
  18. Mesomelic dysplasia
      a) type NIEVERGELT
      b) type LANGER (probable homozygous dyschondrosteosis)

c) type ROBINOW
   d) type RHEINARDT
   e) Others
19. Acromesomelic dysplasia
20. Cleido-cranial dysplasia
21. LARSEN syndrome
22. Oto-palato-digital syndrome

B) Identifiable in later life

1. Hypochondroplasia
2. Dyschondrosteosis
3. Metaphyseal chondrodysplasia type JANSEN
4. Metaphyseal chondrodysplasia type SCHMID
5. Metaphyseal chondrodysplasia type MCKUSICK
6. Metaphyseal chondrodysplasia with exocrine pancreatic insufficiency and cyclic neutropenia
7. Spondylo-metaphyseal dysplasia
   a) type KOZLOWSKI
   b) Other forms
8. Multiple epiphyseal dysplasia
   a) type FAIRBANK
   b) Others
9. Arthro-ophthalmopathy (STICKLER)
10. Pseudo-achondroplasia
    a) Dominant
    b) Recessive
11. Spondylo-epiphyseal tarda
12. Spondylo-epiphyseal dysplasia (other types)
13. DYGGVE-MELCHIOR-CLAUSEN dysplasia
14. Spondylo-epi-metaphyseal dysplasia (several types)
15. Myotonic chondrodysplasia (CATEL-SCHWARTZ-JAMPEL)
16. Parastremmatic dysplasia
17. Tricho-rhino-phalangeal dysplasia
18. Acrodysplasia with retinitis pigmentosa and nephropathy (SALDINO-MAINZER).

This book concerns itself only with the conditions in Group (A) i. e. those manifested at birth. It follows closely the updated nomenclature but conditions such as the oto-palato-digital syndrome have been omitted as their diagnosis may be largely clinical.

Introduction

Just over a decade ago at an International Congress of Pediatric Radiology, the doyen of the meeting was overheard to say "these infantile bone dysplasias all look the same to me." Many others, ourselves included, had the same problem! Since then there has been an explosion of interest in the subject and, with the accumulation of clinical and radiographic data, the features of a number of specific disorders have now been clearly defined. These entities differ widely in their complications and prognosis but they are all heritable conditions with a specific recurrence risk. For these reasons diagnostic accuracy is crucial and in most instances this can now be achieved.

Diagnosis usually depends upon the radiological recognition of a pattern of skeletal change. To recognize this pattern and obtain the maximum information a system and sequence for examining the infant's radiographs must be followed. The majority of diagnostic features are present in (I) the limbs, (II) the thorax and pelvis, (III) the spine, and (IV) the skull. For easier reading we have presented the radiographic features in this order in the text. If after noting and comparing these features the reader is unable to reach a decision then the case probably belongs to an undiagnosable or undelineated category.

Diagnosis is not always easy, but there is little doubt that the problem of skeletal dysplasia in infancy will play an increasing role in modern pediatric radiology. Considerable attention is focused on this topic and trainees in this specialty are expected to have knowledge and a balanced perspective for their examinations. Similarly, the genetic background and potential lethality of many of these disorders is of importance to pediatricians and obstetricians.

We have attempted to produce a concise atlas which contains the relevant information rather than a comprehensive monograph. Wherever possible salient points are discussed in the light of our own practical experience in the Radiology and Genetic departments of the University of Cape Town Medical School. With four exceptions the illustrations are also derived from these sources. We have aimed at simplicity and clarity, and the references which have been selected refer to up-to-date reviews or articles. For further reading a list of relevant articles and monographs is given in the appendix.

The general layout of the appropriate sections of the recently updated (1977) Paris Nomenclature for Constitutional Disorders of Bone has been followed, and in accordance with modern trends we have preferred the term "dysplasia" to that of "dwarfism." Similarly, eponyms have been retained only when they are hallowed by time or where they are in everyday usage.

Chapter 1
Clinical and Genetic Evaluation of the Neonate with Skeletal Dysplasia

In the skeletal dysplasias a firm diagnosis is essential for meaningful prognostication and effective genetic counseling. This is usually dependent upon the accumulation and correlation of information from a number of sources and as several of the skeletal dysplasias are potentially lethal the opportunity to obtain objective evidence may be fleeting. In these circumstances, a full clinical, genetic, and radiographic evaluation is imperative.

Clinical Evaluation

Many of the skeletal dysplasia syndromes present as short-limbed dwarfism and can be grouped according to the prognosis in the perinatal period:

1. Lethal
Achondrogenesis
Thanatophoric dysplasia
Asphyxiating thoracic dysplasia (severe neonatal type)
Short rib-polydactyly syndromes
Campomelic dysplasia
Homozygous achondroplasia

2. Sometimes lethal
Chondroectodermal dysplasia
Chondrodysplasia punctata (rhizomelic type)
Diastrophic dysplasia
Metatropic dysplasia
Osteogenesis imperfecta congenita
Hypophosphatasia (infantile type)
Osteopetrosis—precocious form

3. Not usually lethal
Achondroplasia
Spondyloepiphyseal dysplasia congenita
Mesomelic dysplasia

Certain clinical features are of value as diagnostic indicators, although it must be emphasized that these are neither consistent nor specific:

1. Caput membranaceum
Osteogenesis imperfecta congenita
Hypophosphatasia

2. Cleft palate
Diastrophic dysplasia
Campomelic dysplasia
Spondyloepiphyseal dysplasia congenita

3. Contractures (club foot, flexed digits, etc.)
Diastrophic dysplasia
Chondrodysplasia punctata (sometimes)
Metatropic dysplasia
Campomelic dysplasia
Mesomelic dysplasia—Nievergelt form

4. Supernumerary digits
Short rib-polydactyly syndromes
Asphyxiating thoracic dysplasia
Chondro-ectodermal dysplasia

Genetic Evaluation

Genetic investigations are now an integral component of clinical practice. The neonatal skeletal dysplasias all have a genetic basis and a working knowledge of fundamental concepts concerning the major patterns of inheritance is essential for their understanding and investigation.

A detailed family history will often indicate or at least provide a clue to the probable mode of transmission of a particular disorder. In turn, this information can be used to support or refute a clinical or radiographic diagnosis. For practical purposes the only forms of inheritance likely to be encountered in the neonatal skeletal dysplasias are autosomal dominant and autosomal recessive. In the former case, the condition is handed down from generation to generation and an affected individual has an even chance of transmitting the abnormal gene to each of his or her children. In the latter, clinically normal parents each carry a gene for a particular disorder which only becomes manifest in those of their offspring who receive both of these genes. For any further offspring of this particular couple the risk of the recurrence of the disorder is one in four for every subsequent pregnancy.

This brief account is an oversimplification as many other factors enter into the situation, such as new mutation and genetic heterogeneity. Nevertheless, the following facts should be adduced in every case:

a) Any brothers or sisters with the condition? (i.e., affected siblings and normal parents would suggest autosomal recessive inheritance)

b) Any other affected kin? (i.e., an affected parent would suggest autosomal dominant inheritance)

c) Parents' ages? (i.e., in a sporadic case advanced paternal age would be evidence in favor of new dominant mutation)

d) Parental consanguinity? (i.e., if the parents are related to each other, the condition is likely to be autosomal recessive)

Atypical or undiagnosable neonatal skeletal dysplasias are frequently encountered. With the accumulation of data a number of these have been elevated to syndrome status. Information concerning the probable genetic background provides important clues to their pathogenesis and permits the estimation of recurrence risks.

Genetic Counseling and Antenatal Diagnosis

If a couple has produced a child with a skeletal dysplasia, they will wish to know the prognosis for life and health and the likelihood of recurrence at any future pregnancy. If an accurate diagnosis has been reached this information can be provided. In this situation it is the genetic counselor's duty to ensure that the parents have a clear understanding of the implications of the condition and of the magnitude of the risks of recurrence. He is also obliged to point out the options that are available; these may include avoidance of pregnancy, therapeutic termination, and antenatal diagnosis.

At present amniocentesis is the method of choice in this rapidly expanding field of prenatal diagnosis. In this procedure a needle is passed through the abdominal wall into the uterus and a specimen of amniotic fluid is withdrawn. This is usually undertaken at the 14th to 16th week after conception. Fetal cells can be obtained by centrifugation of this fluid and cultured for the investigation of their cytogenetic status and metabolic activity. By this means certain fetal abnormalities can be recognized sufficiently early to permit selective termination. However, the chromosomes are normal in the skeletal dysplasias and in the majority, the underlying biochemical defects have not been identified. For these reasons, with the exception of hypophosphatasia, they cannot be diagnosed by amniocentesis.

In fetoscopy an optic system attached to a needle is inserted into the gravid uterus. In this way direct visualization of the fetus is possible. Structural defects such as limb-shortening are visible and this technique, therefore, holds considerable promise for the antenatal recognition of the skeletal dysplasias. There are, however, technical problems in fetoscopy and so far it has not found a place in routine practice.

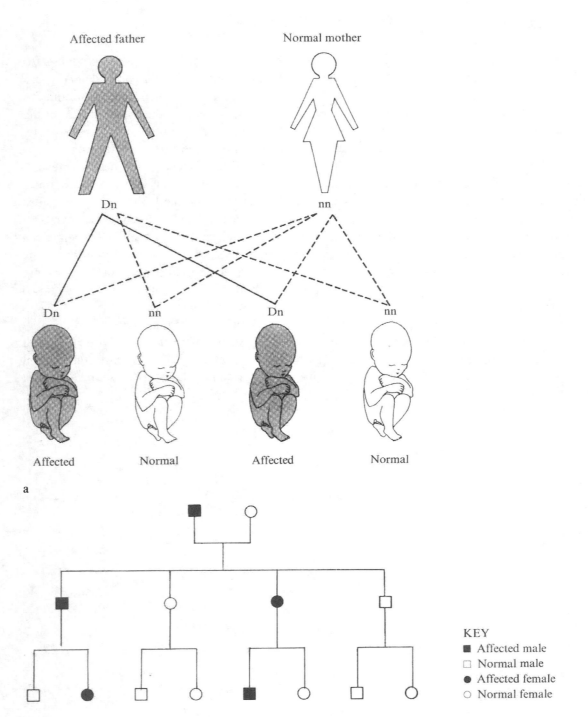

Fig. 1-1. (a) Mechanism of autosomal dominant inheritance. An individual with the abnormal gene, labeled (Dn), will have the clinical features of the disorder. (b) Pedigree of a family with an autosomal dominant disorder such as achondroplasia. Any individual with the abnormality has an even chance of producing an affected child at each episode of procreation, irrespective of the sex of the parent or offspring. The gene is transmitted from generation to generation and approximately equal numbers of males and females are affected

Chapter 1 (Figs. 1-a, b)

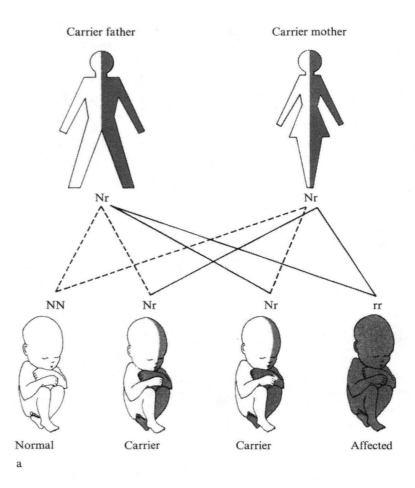

KEY
- ■ Affected male
- □ Normal male
- ● Affected female
- ○ Normal female
- ◨ Clinically normal carrier male
- ◐ Clinically normal carrier female
- / Deceased

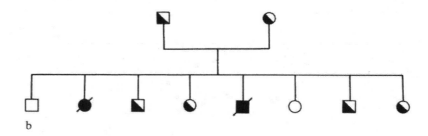

Fig. 1-2. (a) Mechanism of autosomal recessive inheritance. The unaffected parents have an abnormal gene (r) paired with a normal gene (N). When they reproduce, there is a 1 in 4 risk that any child will receive both abnormal genes and thus manifest the disorder. The offspring receiving one normal and one abnormal gene will be clinically normal carriers (heterozygotes) in the same way as their parents. (b) Pedigree of a kindred with an autosomal recessive disorder such as achondrogenesis. The parents are normal but there is a 1 in 4 chance that any offspring, irrespective of sex, will be affected

Chapter 2
Radiographic Techniques

Antenatal Radiology

It is of the utmost importance that radiation to the unborn is avoided wherever possible and the use of ultrasonography is rightly preferred for assessing fetal maturity and position. When there is the possibility of skeletal dysplasia, however, radiography is superior to all other methods in the third trimester. The authors do not associate themselves with the indiscriminate use of radiography and recognize that this is an emotive subject. Nevertheless, the welfare of the mother, both obstetrically and psychologically, and the future of the fetus require that an accurate antenatal diagnosis be made without danger to either of them.

A radiographer can be trained to assess the position of the fetus by abdominal palpation in order to place the mother in the relevant oblique position, with the back of the fetus close to the film. Figure 2-1 shows the prone oblique technique.

1. The prone oblique view gives the most satisfactory results. The fetus is close to the film, its skeleton does not overlap the maternal spine, and the maternal lumbar muscles filter off some of the softer radiation. The use of a "low" kVp technique, 60–70 kVp, as against the more commonly used "high" 120 kVp gives enhanced clarity of the fetal bones. The highest mA and the shortest possible time should be used to give an exposure in the region of 200–250 mAs (3 phase generator). RUSSELL (1973) and FISHER and RUSSELL (1975) have shown that by using this low kVp technique the approximate fetal dose is 0.07 rad, with no increased radiation to the fetus as compared to the more frequently used high kVp techniques. High speed film and fast screens are readily available and are important for satisfactory results. The conventional film-focus distance is 100 cms.

2. The use of a standard abdominal compression band is the second most important factor. Prior to its application an explanation must be given to the gravid patient to allay apprehension. She must also empty her bladder. The technique is quite safe; it not only displaces maternal tissues thus reducing scatter and radiation, but also immobilizes the fetus during exposure. The exposure should be made at deep inspiration so that the fetus is displaced downward into the pelvis.

3. Lead rubber sheeting is placed on the x-ray table next to the maternal abdomen. This helps to reduce scatter from the table-top and thus reduces blackening of the periphery of the radiograph. In some circumstances, depending upon the x-ray unit, additional tube filtration may be necessary.

4. The lateral is an alternative position for demonstrating fetal abnormality. The fetal back should be nearest the film and the maternal back is extended by keeping the legs and arms straight. Exposures are made at approximately 70 kVp and 100 mAs with three-phase equipment. We have found the lateral position more useful for studying the epiphyseal centres for fetal maturity, when ultrasound is not available. We prefer, however, the prone oblique position for routine use; occasionally both projections will be needed.

Ultrasonography

At present ultrasonography is not superior to conventional radiology in demonstrating skeletal dysplasias in the last trimester of pregnancy but gross abnormalities such as anencephaly, hydrocephaly, and spinal dysraphism (KOSSOFF et al., 1974) can be detected by this method. When hydramnios is present the increased amniotic fluid makes ultrasonic definition of the fetus relatively easy. A standard conventional grey-scale unit is employed and the routine examination is conducted in the supine position using a 2.5 MHz transducer. The increased limb soft tissues and relatively large head that are associated with micromelic conditions such as thanatophoric dwarfism have been detected (CREMIN and SHAFF, 1977) (Fig. 2-2a, b), as has the "boneless skull" of hypophosphatasia (RUDD et al., 1976).

Amniography and Fetography

These methods have only a small part to play in the diagnosis of fetal skeletal abnormality. Delineation of the fetal limbs may be made easier in the second trimester and in mothers who have had previous genetic problems of this type, amniography may be justified (GOLBUS et al., 1977). Although hydramnios is a frequent accompaniment of many skeletal dysplasias, its sudden development in the third trimester may be an indication for amniography to exclude fetal foregut anomalies.

Prior to amniography the placenta is located by palpation or ultrasonography. After the patient has emptied her bladder suprapubic amniocentesis is undertaken, using a BECTON-DICKINSON Longdwell cannula-overneedle, 30–40 ml (less in the second trimester) of fluid are withdrawn and replaced by an equal amount of a water-soluble contrast media of the meglumine type (such as Urografin 76 or Renografin 60). Films are taken after 1 h and 12 h to demonstrate the passage of contrast medium through the alimentary tract.

Fetography may be useful to show spinal defects that have an exterior component. Six ml of an oily substance such as Iodophendylate (Myodil or Pantopaque) is injected into the amniotic sac. This medium is absorbed by the vernix caseosa coating the fetus and gives a vivid outline of the fetal contours. After 36 weeks maturity absorption is appreciably diminished but, nevertheless, increased fetal soft tissues which occur in hydropic infants, such as thanatophoric dwarfs, can be demonstrated (Fig. 2-2). Complications such as premature labor or fetal injury are uncommon when the plastic cannula technique is used (SHAFF, 1977).

Postnatal Radiography

It is of utmost importance that all stillborn infants and neonates dying in the puerperium should be studied radiographically to establish an exact diagnosis. In this way RYAN and KOZLOWSKI (1971) demonstrated an appreciable number of skeletal defects which might otherwise have been undetected. The following methods are in use:

1. Term or near-term infants
Double emulsion, medium-speed film, used in conjunction with high-definition intensifying screens. Average exposure factors at 110 cms FFD, small tube focus (in region of 0.6 mm) are 40 kVp and 6 mAs.

2. Localized views of extremities and infants under 24 eeks
Nonscreen mammography film (fine grain, high-definition) which is envelope-packed for automatic processing at 110 cms FFD. Exposure factors are 35 kVp and 100 mAs.

Anteroposterior and lateral projections are used, the deceased infant being immobilized against the cassette with adhesive tape. Both the above methods have their merits; high contrast in the former but increased definition in the latter. When assessing bony maturity it must be remembered that many stillborn infants are premature.

Examination of the Prenatal Radiograph

The radiographs must be examined systematically if the maximum diagnostic information is to be obtained. For the fetus we suggest varying the order of the examination, outlined for the postnatal infant in the previous chapter, to spine, pelvis, and thorax, skull, and limbs. The axial skeleton is usually easily recognizable, so note the presence and shape of the vertebrae and the general curvature of the spine.

Next assess the pelvis for the shape of the iliac wings and acetabular roofs, and the ribs for appearance and anomalies.

Examine the skull for size and degree of ossification and the presence of vault defects.

The tubular skeleton is often difficult to evaluate *in utero*. The actual presence of all bones must be noted. The size, shape, and texture of the bones, the appearance of metaphyses, maturation of epiphyses (calcaneus ± 26 weeks, talus ± 28 weeks, and lower femora ± 36 weeks), and the configuration of the extremities must be considered. Errors in evaluating the length of the limb bones are easily made if they are only seen obliquely or end-on.

Multidisciplinary Evaluation

Radiographic studies are the most important component of the multidisciplinary approach to the diagnosis of infantile skeletal dysplasias. There are many pitfalls in the assessment of these conditions and the comments made by Prof. J.W. SPRANGER at the meeting of the 1969 European Society of Pediatric Radiologists (Warsaw) still hold true today:
a) Do not diagnose from a single sign, diagnosis must be made from a pattern.
b) Never diagnose from a single site, a skeletal survey is necessary.
c) Have patience if you cannot make the diagnosis in infancy, the pattern may take time to evolve.
d) Lastly, do not publish too early as a single case may only add to the confusion.

Postmortem Staining Techniques

Although it is of little practical value in the evaluation of skeletal dysplasias, the technique of staining with 0.5% silver nitrate solution (Fig. 2-3a, b, c) after fixation in formaldehyde shows to advantage the development of the human skeleton, and the nonspecificity of marginal spicules (seen at the 14th–16th week of development). The larger infants have to be flayed to allow diffusion of silver salt through to the bones (Fig. 2-4). The resultant radiographs show improved bony definition but are of little advantage over good conventional techniques unless the details of smaller bones (such as those of the hand) are required for study.

References

Cremin, B. J., Shaff, M. I.: Ultrasonic diagnosis of thanatophoric dwarfism in utero. *Radiology* **124**, 479 (1977).
Cremin, B. J., Shaff, M. I.: Foetal skeletal abnormalities demonstrated by radiology. *(unpublished material)*.
Fisher, A. S., Russell, J. S. B.: Radiography in Obstetrics. London-Boston: Butterworths 1975.
Golbus, M. S., Hall, B. D., Filly, R. A., Poskanzer, L. B.: Prenatal diagnosis of achondrogenesis. Pediatr. **91**, 464 (1977).
Kossoff, G., Garrett, W. J., Radovanovich, G.: Grey scale echography in obstetrics and gynaecology. Aust. Radiol. **18**, 63 (1974).
Kozlowski, K., Maroteaux, P., Silverman, F., Kaufmann, H., Spranger, J.: Classification des dysplasies osseuses. Table ronde. Ann. Radiol. (Paris) **12** (11—12), 1007 (1969).
Rudd, N. L., Miskin, M., Hoar, D. I., Benzie, R., Doran, T. A.: Prenatal diagnosis of hypophosphatasia. N. Engl. J. Med. **295**, 146 (1976).
Russell, J. S. B.: Radiology in Obstetrics and Antenatal Paediatrics. London: Butterworths 1973.
Ryan, J. F., Kozlowski, K.: Radiography in stillborn infants. Aust. Radiol. **15**, 213 (1971).
Shaff, M. I.: Foetal complications in amniography. Br. J. Radiol. **50**, 8, 41 (1977).

Chapter 2 (Figs. 2-1/2-a, b)

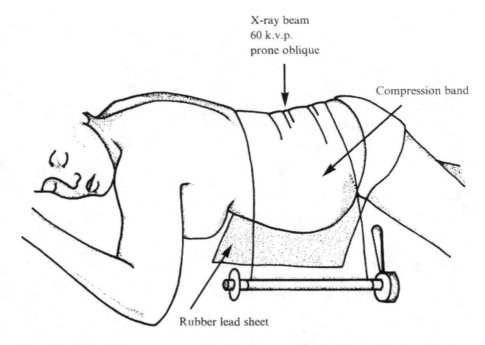

Fig.2-1. Prone oblique position demonstrating the radiographic technique

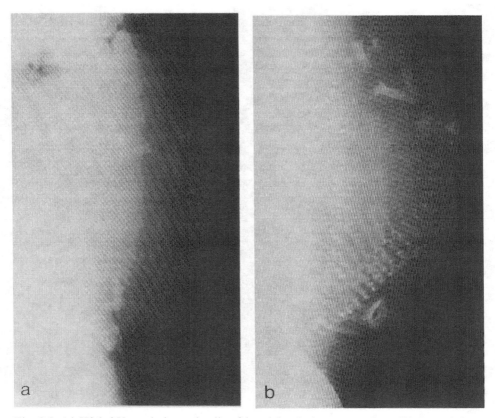

Fig. 2-2. (a) High kVp technique, details of bone dysplasia are not clear. (b) Same infant, low kVp technique, showing features of thanatophoric dwarfism

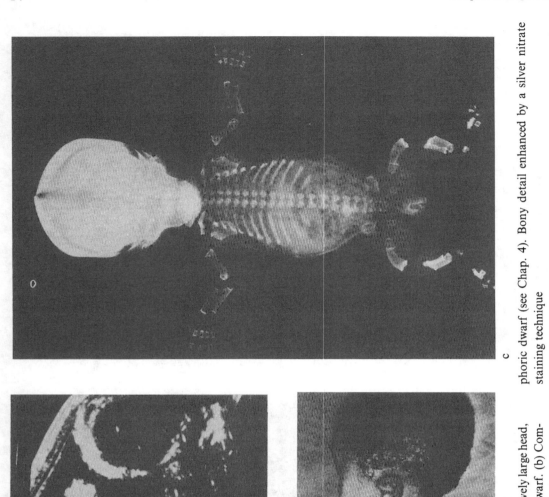

Fig. 2-3 (a) Ultrasonic image of the short, fat limbs, relatively large head, and general hydropic appearance of a thanatophoric dwarf. (b) Comparison of the actual physical appearance after delivery. (c) Thanatophoric dwarf (see Chap. 4). Bony detail enhanced by a silver nitrate staining technique

Chapter 2 (Figs. 2-4/2-5/2-6) 15

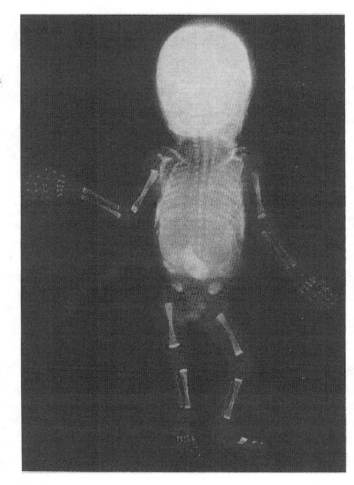

Fig. 2-4. 14-week fetus showing bones stained by silver nitrate

Fig. 2-5. Magnified view of the lower limbs of an 11-week fetus showing the non-specific scalloped appearance in the early stages of chondro-osseous development

Fig. 2-6. 14-week fetus showing further maturation

Fig. 2-4

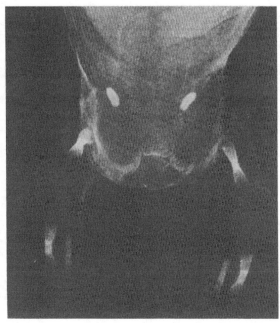

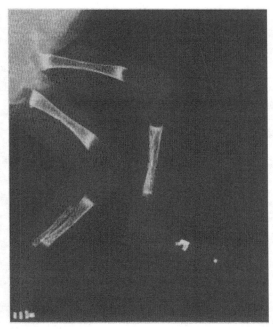

Fig. 2-5

Fig. 2-6

Chapter 3
Achondrogenesis

There has been semantic confusion concerning the use of the term achondrogenesis as it was initially employed by GREBE (1953) to describe an unrelated, nonlethal form of short-limbed dwarfism. The eponym "Grebe syndrome" is now applied to this entity, while "achondrogenesis" pertains to the lethal condition which forms the subject of this chapter. The nosological situation has been further confused by the recognition of subtypes of achondrogenesis and by the application of overlapping numeric designations.

Classification of Achondrogenesis

Achondrogenesis Type I Parenti-Fraccaro (previously type 1 A)
Achondrogenesis Type II Langer-Saldino (previously type 1 B)

Type I and type II forms of achondrogenesis are generally accepted as separate entities, although the difference between them is essentially radiological. Both forms are equally lethal but the bony dysplasia of the limbs is most severe in type I, in which development is only rudimentary. The features of achondrogenesis have been reviewed by WIEDEMANN et al. (1974), YANG et al. (1974), and Ho and TAN (1976). About 40 cases have now been reported.

Clinical Manifestations

Affected infants are almost always stillborn. The combination of a relatively large head, severe micromelia, a prominent abdomen, and a squat trunk are easily recognized, and the diagnosis can be strongly suspected on a clinical basis, pending radiographic confirmation.

Radiographic Features

The skeleton is severely underossified with defective development of many components. The main radiographic features are summarized in Table 1.
　　The main diagnostic differences are that in type I there are marked changes in the limbs and pelvis and although the vertebral bodies are virtually unossified, the posterior elements are present. In type II the limbs are more well formed while spinal changes may include absence of lumbar vertebrae.
　　These distinctive radiographic changes permit intrauterine diagnosis when high quality radiographs are obtained during the third trimester.

Table 1

	Type I	Type II
Limbs	Gross shortening and irregularity, to extent of rudimentary ossicles	Changes less gross but severe shortening with metaphyseal widening and cupping present
Thorax	Thin ribs with flared anterior ends, possible fractures	Ribs relatively short and stubby
Pelvis	Very poorly ossified iliac bones, sacrum and pubic bones absent	Iliac bones small but moderately well ossified, deficient sacrum and pubic bones
Spine	Deficient ossification of vertebral bodies from absence to small ossified centre	Nonossification of some vertebral bodies, especially in lumbar region
Skull	Variable degree of vault underossification	Good ossification of vault

Comment

Both types of achondrogenesis are inherited as autosomal recessives. There is, therefore, a one in four risk of recurrence for each subsequent child of parents who have produced an affected infant (Housten et al., 1972). Although radiographic intrauterine diagnosis is possible, this procedure cannot be undertaken sufficiently early to permit selective abortion.

Harris et al. (1972) and Lauder et al. (1976) described siblings with achondrogenesis and fractures, while Verma et al. (1975) report a lethal short-limbed dwarfism in a consanguineous kindred under the title "achondrogenesis type III." The relationship of these entities with classic achondrogenesis is uncertain. Kozlowski et al. (1977) reported a further series of cases of lethal dwarfism and proposed further sub-categorisation. It must be emphasized that these various forms of achondrogenesis are not entirely distinct and that no classification is yet definitive.

References

Grebe, H.: Die Achondrogenesis, ein einfach rezessives Erbmerkmal. Folia Hered. et Pathol. (Milano) 2, 23 (1953).
Harris, R., Patton, I. T., Barson, A. J.: Pseudoachondrogenesis with fractures. Clin. Genet. 3, 435 (1972).
Ho, N.-K., Tan, G.: Achondrogenesis, a clinical and radiological report. Aust. Radiol. 20, 165 (1976).
Houston, C. S., Awen, C. F., Kent, H. P.: Fatal neonatal dwarfism. J. Can. Assoc. Radiol. 23, 45 (1973).
Kozlowski, K., Mosel, J., Morris, L., Ryan, J., Collins, F., Van Vliet, P., Woolnough, H.: Neonatal death dwarfism (report of 17 cases). Aust. Radiol., 21, 164 (1977)
Lauder, I., Ellis, H. A., Ashcroft, T., Burridge, A.: Achondrogenesis type I. A familial subvariant? Arch. Dis. Child. 51, 550 (1976).
Verma, I. C., Bhargava, S., Agarwal, A.: An autosomal recessive form of lethal chondrodystrophy with severe thoracic narrowing, rhizoacromelic type of micromelia, polydactyly and genital anomalies. Birth Defects 11/6, 167 (1975).
Wiedemann, H. R., Remagen, W., Hienz, H. A.: Achondrogenesis within the scope of connately manifested generalised skeletal dysplasias. Z. Kinderheilk. 116/4, 223 (1974).
Yang, S. S., Brougn, A. J., Garewal, G. S., Bernstein, J.: Two types of inheritable lethal achondrogenesis. J. Paediatr. 85/6, 796 (1974).

Chapter 3 (Figs. 3-a, b) 19

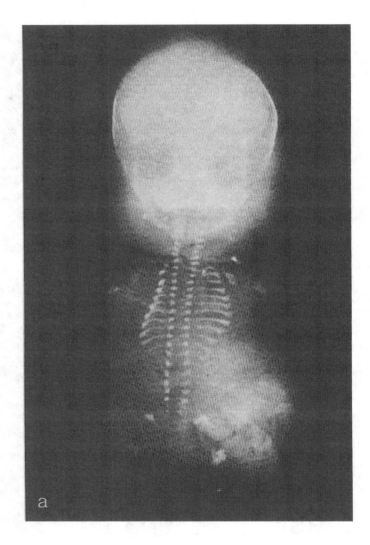

Type I

Fig. 3-1. (a) Stillborn infant with grossly deficient ossification of the limbs, only small spicules of bone being present. The pubic bones and vertebral bodies have not ossified but the posterior components of the vertebra have developed.

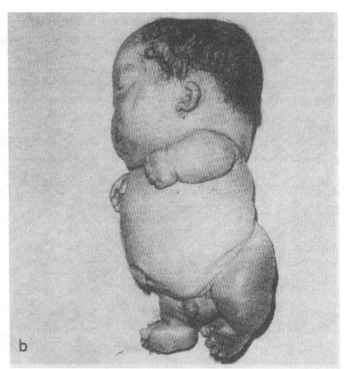

Fig. 3-1. (b) Photograph of the above infant demonstrating the relatively large head, squat trunk and severe micromelia

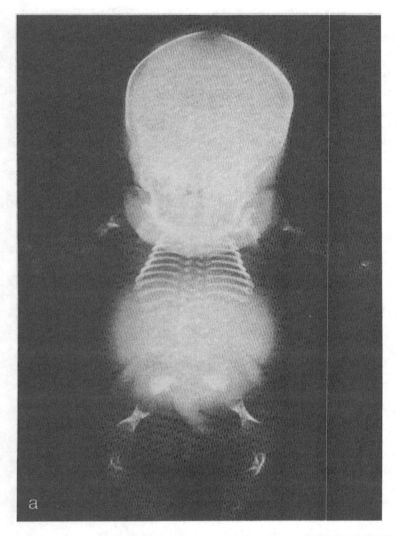

Type II

Fig. 3-2. (a) AP, after stillbirth, illustrating the limb and spine changes. The iliac bones are small but ossified while the pubic bones and lumbar spine are absent. (b) *In utero* radiograph at 30 weeks. The tubular bones are short, with concave extremities; ossification of the lower spine is deficient. (c) Lateral, showing micromelia, short ribs and defective ossification of the lower vertebrae

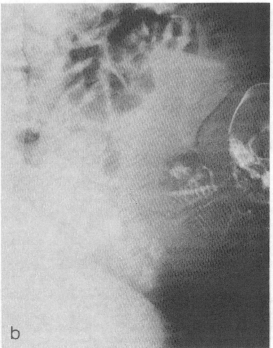

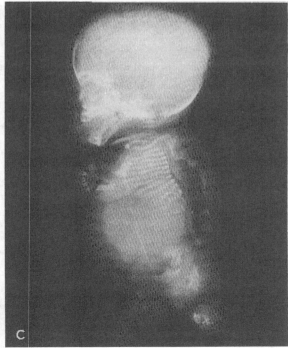

Chapter 4
Thanatophoric Dysplasia

Thanatophoric dysplasia was differentiated from achondroplasia by MAROTEAUX et al. (1967). The name is derived from the Greek term for death-bearing. This disorder, which has well-defined radiographic features, is the commonest form of fatal neonatal dwarfism.

Clinical Manifestations

The most obvious clinical features are marked limb-shortening with a normal sized trunk, in which the bulging abdomen contrasts with the narrow thorax. The head is comparatively large, with a prominent forehead and a depressed nasal bridge. The majority of affected infants are stillborn or die within hours of birth and the few that survive for a matter of days eventually succumb to respiratory failure (MOIR and KOZLOWSKI, 1976).

Radiographic Features

I. Limbs. Distinctive changes are present in the tubular bones. The long bones are short and slightly bowed. The shortening is predominantly rhizomelic and the bowing is most marked in the femora, which frequently take on a curved "telephone receiver" appearance. The metaphyses show widening, cupping, and irregularity; no ossification centers are visible in the distal femoral or proximal tibial epiphyseal regions. The only ossification centers which are seen consistently are those in the calcaneus and talus.

The short tubular bones of the hands and feet are maldeveloped, and the first metacarpals and metatarsals are shorter and wider than the others. The proximal phalanges show distal central beaking and the middle and distal phalanges are markedly shortened.

II. Thorax and Pelvis. The anteroposterior diameter of the chest is narrowed and the ribs are short with cupping and flaring of their anterior ends. The clavicles are normal but the scapulae are shortened in their vertical and horizontal diameters with squaring of their lower borders. The pelvis is also shortened, with squaring of the iliac wings, which have horizontal and slightly spiculated lower margins.

III. Spine. The notable characteristic is lack of ossification of the vertebral bodies which increases craniocaudally, so that the bodies are flattened or disklike. The posterior aspects of the vertebrae, including the pedicles, are relatively unaffected. Slight progressive caudal narrowing of the lower lumbar interpedicular spaces may occur. In the lateral projection the disklike shape of the bodies is a prominent feature. The reduced vertebral body height together with the less affected posterior vertebral components, produces a characteristic "H" or inverted "U" appearance in the AP projection which is seen most predominantly in the lumbar region.

IV. Skull. The skull shows variable enlargement of the calvarium with shortening of the base and involvement of the foramen magnum.

Comment

The salient radiographic features may be demonstrated antenatally (CAMPBELL, 1971). Apart from the micromelia difficulty may be experienced in identifying the limb configuration and in these cases the disklike lateral and H-shaped frontal appearance of the vertebrae can be a valuable aid to diagnosis. The relatively large head and the short and podgy limbs can also be recognized ultrasonically (Chap. 2, Fig. 2) (CREMIN and SHAFF, 1977).

There is controversy concerning the etiology of thanatophoric dysplasia but it is probably nongenetic with a low recurrence risk (PENA and GOODMAN, 1973). Nevertheless, antenatal recognition is important, as the bulging calvarium may cause cephalopelvic disproportion and obstruct normal delivery (THOMPSON and PARMLEY, 1971).

The clinical resemblance of thanatophoric dysplasia to achondroplasia has been a source of much confusion and misdiagnosis is not at all uncommon (HARRIS and PATTON, 1971; BERGSTROM et al., 1972). The characteristic radiographic features permit, however, accurate distinction between these entities (GIEDION, 1968; LANGER et al., 1969; KAUFMAN et al., 1970; SALDINO, 1971; NISSENBAUM et al., 1977). Histologically there has also been confusion as several studies on neonatal "achondroplasia" have in fact been performed on thanatophoric dwarfs (RIMOIN et al., 1973).

The clinical and radiographic stigmata of homozygous or doubly affected achondroplastic neonates are similar to those of thanatophoric dysplasia, but as the parents in this latter situation must both be achondroplasts, diagnostic problems do not arise.

A "cloverleaf" skull or "Kleeblattschädel" is due to premature synostosis of cranial sutures resulting in a trefoil configuration with upward and lateral bulging of the calvarium. It has been reported in a number of infants with thanatophoric dysplasia (BLOOMFIELD, 1970; PARTINGTON et al., 1971; YOUNG et al., 1973; INNACCONE and GERLINI, 1974). The etiologic relationship of these skeletal anomalies is uncertain but it is possibly that forms of thanatophoric dysplasia with and without these skull changes are separate entities. It must be emphasized, however, that the cloverleaf skull can also occur in isolation or as a component of a variety of other syndromes (TEMTAMY et al., 1975). Radiographic antenatal detection of this skull anomaly is important for the obstetric management of the patient.

References

BERGSTROM, K., GUSTAVON, K. H., JORULF, H.: Thanatophoric dwarfism: diagnosis in utero. Aust. Radiol. **16**, 156 (1972).
BLOOMFIELD, J. A.: Cloverleaf skull and thanatophoric dwarfism. Aust. Radiol. **14**, 429 (1970).
CAMPBELL, R. E.: Thanatophoric dwarfism in utero: a case report. Am. J. Roentgenol. **112**, 198 (1971).
CREMIN, B. J., SHAFF, M. I.: Ultrasonic diagnosis of thanatophoric dwarfism in utero. Radiology **124**, 479 (1977).
GIEDION, A.: Thanatophoric dwarfism. Helv. Paediat. Acta **23**, 175 (1968).
HARRIS, R., PATTON, J. T.: Achondroplasia and thanatophoric dwarfism in the newborn. Clin. Genet. **2**, 61 (1971).
IANNACCONE, G., GERLINI, G.: The so-called "cloverleaf skull syndrome." Pediatr. Radiol. **2**, 175 (1974).
KAUFMAN, R. L., RIMOIN, D. L., McALISTER, W. H., KISSANE, I. M.: Thanatophoric dwarfism. Am. J. Dis. Child. **120**, 53 (1970).
LANGER, L. O., JR., SPRANGER, J. W., GREINACHER, I., HERDAMN, R. C.: Thanatophoric dwarfism. A condition confused with achondroplasia in the neonate, with brief comments on achondrogenesis and homozygous achondroplasia. Radiology **92**, 285 (1969).
MAROTEAUX, P., LAMY, M., ROBERT, J. M.: Le nanisme thanatophore. Presse Méd. **75**, 2519 (1967).

References

Moir, D. H., Kozlowski, K.: Long survival in thanatophoric dwarfism. Pediatr. Radiol. **5**, 123 (1976).

Nissenbaum, M., Chung, S. M. K., Rosenberg, H. K., Buck, B. E.: Thanatophoric Dwarfism. Two case reports and survey of the literature. Clin. Pediat. **16**, 690 (1977).

Partington, M. W., Gonzales-Crussi, F., Khakee, S. G., Wollin, D. G.: Cloverleaf skull and thanatophoric dwarfism. Report of four cases, two in the same sibship. Arch. Dis. Child. **46**, 656 (1971).

Pena, S. D. J., Goodman, H. D.: The genetics of thanatophoric dwarfism. Pediatrics **51**, 104 (1973).

Rimoin, D. L., McAlister, W. H., Saldino, R. M., Hall, J. G.: Histologic Appearances of Some Types of Congenital Dwarfism. Progress in Pediatric Radiology, Intrinsic Diseases of Bone, Vol. IV, p. 67. Basel: Karger 1973.

Saldino, R. M.: Lethal short-limbed dwarfism: achondrogenesis and thanatophoric dwarfism. Am. J. Roentgenol. **112**, 185 (1971).

Temtamy, S. A., Shoukry, A. S., Fayad, I., El Meligy, M. R.: Limb malformations in the cloverleaf skull anomaly. Birth Defects **11/2**, 247 (1975).

Thompson, B. H., Parmley, T. H.: Obstetric features of thanatophoric dwarfism. Am. J. Obstet. Gynaecol. **109**, 396 (1971).

Young, R. S., Pocharzevsky, Leonicas, J. C., Wexler, I. B., Ratner, H.: Thanatophoric dwarfism and cloverleaf skull ("Kleeblattschädel"). Radiology **106**, 401 (1973).

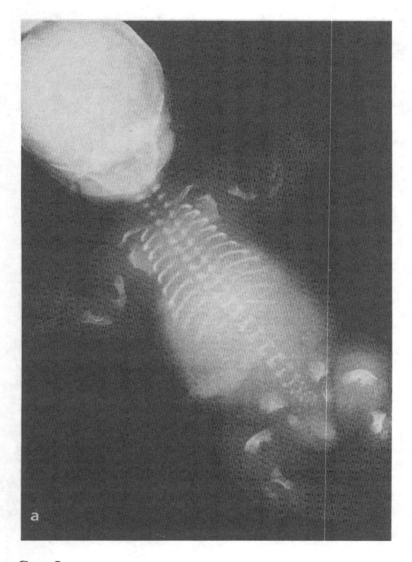

Case I

Fig. 4-1. (a) AP projection. The tubular bones are short and curved, and the femora have a "telephone-receiver" configuration. Deficient ossification of the vertebral bodies produces an "H" appearance. The ribs are short and the scapulae are undercut

Chapter 4 (Figs. 4-1/4-2)

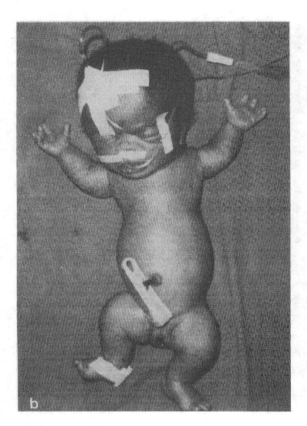
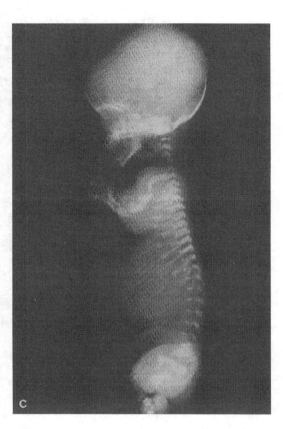

Fig. 4-1. (b) Stillborn infant. The relatively large head, depressed nasal bridge, constricted thorax, and short limbs are typical but nonspecific features. (c) Lateral projection. The vertebral bodies appear disklike and ribs are shortened

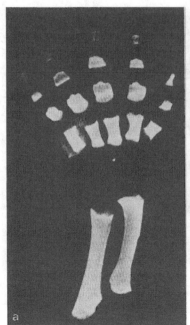
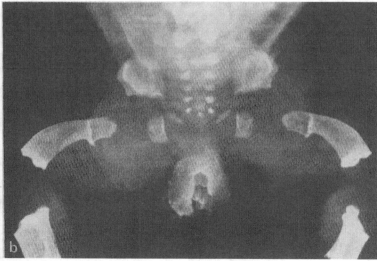

Case II

Fig. 4-2. (a) Silver nitrate staining of hand and forearm. For description see text. (b) Details of pelvis and lower limbs illustrated by staining technique (p. 11)

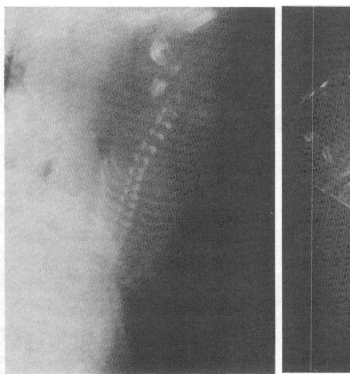

Case III

Fig. 4-3. *In utero*, prone oblique radiograph showing short ribs, typical "H" vertebrae and curvature of femora. The fetus is aged at least 32 weeks as an abdominal fat line is visible

Case IV

Fig. 4-4. Fetoamniograph; the contrast material (myodil) which outlines the skin shows the hydropic appearance (there is also water-soluble, contrast medium in the intestines). The short "telephone receiver" shaped femur is arrowed

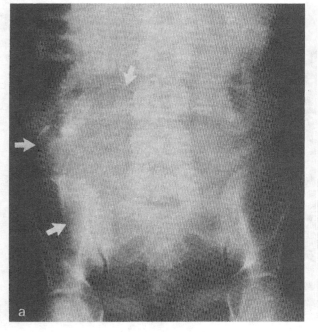
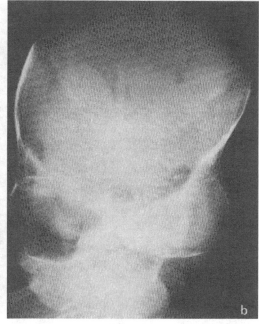

Case V

Fig. 4-5. (a) Short-limbed dwarf with a clover-leaf skull (*arrowed*) in utero. Supine radiograph; a prone oblique projection would have shown the features of thanatophoric dwarfism to better advantage. (b) Trefoil or cloverleaf skull with gross ballooning of cranial vault and middle cranial fossa

Chapter 5
Asphyxiating Thoracic Dysplasia

This condition, described in a pair of siblings by JEUNE et al. (1955), is also known as infantile thoracic dystrophy, thoracopelvicphalangeal dystrophy, and the Jeune syndrome. The stigmata and clinical course are very variable and it is possible that the disorder is heterogeneous (KAUFMANN and KIRKPATRICK, 1974; KOZLOWSKI and MASEL, 1976).

Clinical Manifestations

The main clinical feature is thoracic constriction and an elongated immobile chest. Limb shortening is variable but not marked. Polydactyly is present in about 20% of cases (JEQUIER et al., 1973). There is a wide spectrum of severity but death from respiratory distress occurs in early infancy in the majority of patients. Among the survivors the shape of the chest tends to revert to normal, but renal failure usually supervenes (LANGER, 1968) and few patients reach adulthood (FRIEDMAN et al., 1975).

Radiographic Features

I. Limbs. Shortening of the tubular bones is not usually marked and they are not bowed. Maturation of the femoral capital epiphyses is accelerated and they may be visible in the neonate or in early infancy (CREMIN, 1970). (In the normal child these epiphyses are not seen before the fourth month.)

The hands have no distinctive features at birth but at a later stage the phalanges may show nonspecific, coneshaped epiphyses. These may fuse prematurely to give digital shortening and peripheral dysostosis.

II. Thorax and Pelvis. The most obvious radiographic changes are seen in the chest and pelvis. The anteroposterior diameter of the thorax is markedly reduced and the ribs are short and horizontally placed with cupped or flared anterior ends. The clavicles are often inverted, with a "high handlebar" appearance, while the sternum may show incomplete ossification.

In the pelvis the iliac bones are shortened and their lateral borders are usually rounded rather than squared. The acetabular roof has a trident configuration or three-part irregularity due to lateral spicules and a central spur. This appearance may not be prominent and varies with age, diminishes with growth, and may be indistinguishable from that of chondroectodermal dysplasia.

III. Spine. There are no notable abnormalities.

Comment

Patients who survive infancy tend to outgrow the radiographic changes in their long bones and pelvis. In later life the thoracic changes are variable in degree.

Thoracic constriction is a feature of several other disorders (KOHLER and BABBITT, 1970), while polydactyly occurs in a variety of neonatal dwarfism syndromes (KOZLOWSKI et al., 1972). For these reasons, together with the variability of the stigmata, accurate diagnosis in the newborn may be difficult.

KOZLOWSKI and MASEL (1976) reported a "latent" form of the condition, following their recognition of the typical pelvic changes in two children after radiological studies for an unrelated purpose. Rib-shortening in these patients was slight and they had never experienced respiratory problems. It is debatable whether this disorder is a distinct entity or the result of variable phenotypic expression of the same basic defect.

Several sets of affected siblings with normal parents have been reported and inheritance is probably autosomal recessive, the recurrence risk, therefore, being 25%. Diagnosis *in utero* has been reported (RUSSELL and CHOUKSEY, 1970).

References

CREMIN, B. J.: Infantile thoracic dystrophy. Br. J. Radiol. **43**, 199 (1970).
FRIEDMAN, J. M., KAPLAN, H. G., HALL, J. G.: The Jeune syndrome (asphyxiating thoracic dystrophy) in an adult. Am. J. Med. **59/6**, 857 (1975).
JÉQUIER, J.-C., FAVREAU-ETHIER, M., GRÉGOIRE, H.: Intrinsic Diseases of Bones. Progress in Pediatric Radiology. Thoracic Dysplasia, Vol. IV, p. 184. Basel: Karger 1973.
JEUNE, M., BERAUD, C., CARRON, R.: Dystrophie thoracique asphyxiante de caractère familial. Arch. Fr. Pédiatr. **12**, 886 (1955).
KAUFMANN, H. J., KIRKPATRICK, J. A., JR.: Jeune thoracic dysplasia—a spectrum of disorders? Birth Defects **10/9**, 101 (1974).
KOHLER, E., BABBITT, D. P.: Dystrophic thoraces and infantile asphyxia. Radiology **94**, 55 (1970).
KOZLOWSKI, K., MASEL, J.: Asphyxiating thoracic dystrophy without respiratory distress. Pediat. Radiol. **5**, 30 (1976).
KOZLOWSKI, K., SZMIGIEL, CZ., BARYLAK, A., STOPYROWA, M.: Difficulties in differentiation between chondroectodermal dysplasia (Ellis-van Creveld syndrome) and asphyxiating thoracic dystrophy. Aust. Radiol. **16**, 401 (1972).
LANGER, L. O., JR.: Thoracic-pelvic-phalangeal dystrophy: Asphyxiating thoracic dystrophy of the newborn; infantile thoracic dystrophy. Radiology **91**, 447 (1968).
RUSSELL, J. G. B., CHOUKSEY, S. K.: Asphyxiating thoracic dystrophy. Br. J. Radiol. **43**, 814 (1970).

Chapter 5 (Fig. 5-1a)

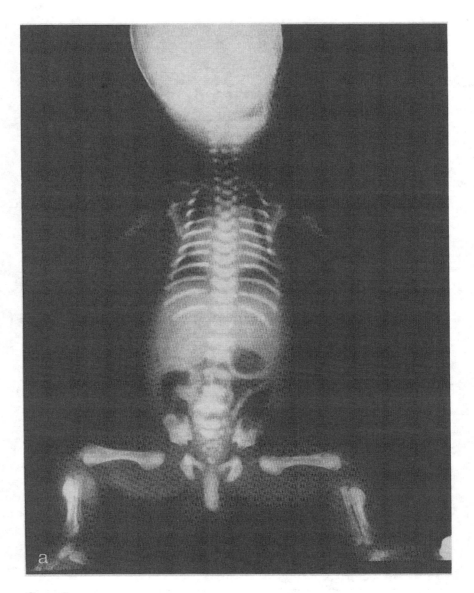

Case I

Fig. 5-1. (a) Radiograph of a newborn infant that died of respiratory distress soon after birth. Characteristic features are marked thoracic constriction, high clavicles, and mild limb-shortening. Acetabular roof, with a central prominence, has a "trident" appearance

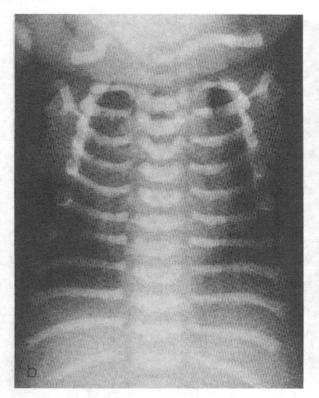
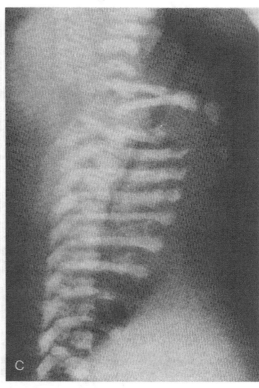
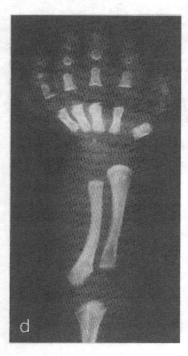

Case I

Fig. 5-1. (b) Chest showing the short, horizontal ribs and high clavicles.
(c) Lateral chest radiograph showing severe rib shortening and deficient ossification of sternum
Fig. 5-1. (d) Forearms shows mild micromelia and is polydactyly (postaxial hexadactyly), an inconsistent feature of the condition

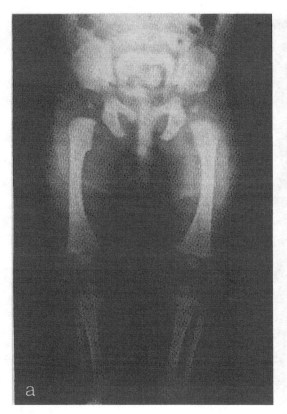
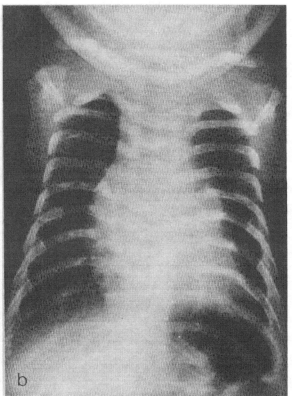

Case II

Fig. 5-2. (a) Pelvis and lower limbs of a 3-month-old infant. Acetabular roof shows some flattening, while ossification of the capital femoral epiphyses is advanced.

Fig. 5-2. (b) Chest at 10 months showing the elongated constricted configuration and the "handlebar" clavicles

Case III

Fig. 5-3. Pelvis of an asymptomatic 5-month-old infant. Clinically and radiologically the chest was normal, but the advanced maturation of the capital femoral epiphyses and the trident acetabular roof are similar to those seen in asphyxiating thoracic dysplasia. This case is included to demonstrate that some of the radiological features may be present in an otherwise normal child. (Courtesy of Dr. J. A. Toland, Dublin)

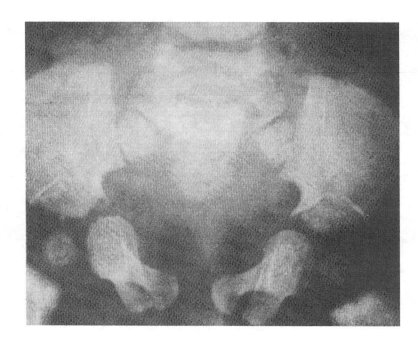

Chapter 6
Chondroectodermal Dysplasia

Ellis and Van Creveld (1940) delineated this syndrome, of which more than 120 cases have now been reported. A large proportion of these have occurred in a consanguineous community, the Amish of Pennsylvania, USA (McKusick et al., 1964; Murdoch and Walker, 1969).

Clinical Manifestations

Limb-shortening in the newborn is most obvious in the forearms and lower legs. Narrowing of the thorax and postaxial polydactyly may be present, and confusion with asphyxiating thoracic dysplasia can arise. Ectodermal anomalies, including abnormalities of the hair, teeth, and nails are important differentiating features. The upper lip may be shortened and fused to the maxillary gingiva.

About 50% of patients have structural cardiac abnormalities, which usually involve the atrial septum, the prognosis being largely determined by the severity of this lesion. In the survivors genu valgum is a common complication. Adult height can be normal.

Radiographic Features

I. Limbs. The limbs tend to be involved more than the trunk, with acromelic micromelia and extra digits. Early ossification of the capital femoral epiphyses has been reported (Kaufmann, 1974).

II. Thorax and Pelvis. Thoracic constriction is not prominent but otherwise the radiographic changes in the pelvis and limbs of the neonate may be virtually indistinguishable from those of asphyxiating thoracic dysplasia. This problem has been discussed in detail by Kozlowski et al. (1972). The features of the trident acetabular roof with its prominent downward medial spur distinguish chondroectodermal dysplasia from achondroplasia, in which the spur tends to be more medially directed (Kaufmann, 1965).

III. Spine and Skull. There are no notable features.

IV. Other Features. In later infancy recognition of the characteristic fusion of the capitate and hamate bones in the carpus, and defective ossification of the medial portion of the proximal femoral metaphysis with subsequent genu valgum permits diagnostic confirmation. Radiological differentiation between asphyxiating thoracic dysplasia and chondroectodermal dysplasia presents no difficulties at this stage.

Comment

Autosomal recessive inheritance is well established but in spite of recurrence risk, *in utero* recognition of the disorder has not been reported. The basic defect is unknown, but disorganised endochondral ossification has been observed in biopsy specimens and amputated digits (BLACKBURN and BELLIVEAU, 1971; LE MAREC et al., 1973).

References

BLACKBURN, M. G., BELLIVEAU, R. E.: Ellis-van Creveld syndrome: A report of previously undescribed anomalies in two siblings. Am. J. Dis. Child. **122**, 267 (1971).
ELLIS, R. W. B., VAN CREVELD, S.: A syndrome characterised by ectodermal dysplasia, polydactyly, chondroplasia, and congenital morbus cordis. Arch. Dis. Child. **15**, 65 (1940).
KAUFMANN, H. J.: The pelvis in the Ellis-van Creveld syndrome. Ann. Radiol. (Paris) **8**, 146 (1965).
KAUFMANN, H. J.: "New" skeletal dysplasias in the newborn: new x-ray finding. Birth Defects **10/12**, 1 (1974).
KOZLOWSKI, K., SZMIGIEL, CZ., BARYLAK, A., STOPYROWA, M.: Difficulties in differentiation between chondroectodermal dysplasia (Ellis-van Creveld syndrome) and asphyxiating thoracic dystrophy. Aust. Radiol. **16**, 401 (1972).
LE MAREC, B., PASSARGE, E., DELLENBACH, P., KERISII, J., SIGNARGOUT, J., FERRAND, B., SENECAL, J.: Les formes néonatales léthales de la dysplasie chondroectodermique: A propos de cinq observations. Ann. Radiol. (Paris) **16**, 19 (1973).
MCKUSICK, V. A., EGELAND, J. A., ELDRIGE, R., KRUSEN, D. E.: Dwarfism in the Amish. The Ellis-van Creveld syndrome. Bull. Johns Hopkins Hosp. **115**, 306 (1964).
MURDOCH, J. L., WALKER, B. A.: Ellis-van Creveld syndrome. Birth Defects **5/4**, 279 (1969).

Chapter 6 (Figs. 6-1a, b, c)

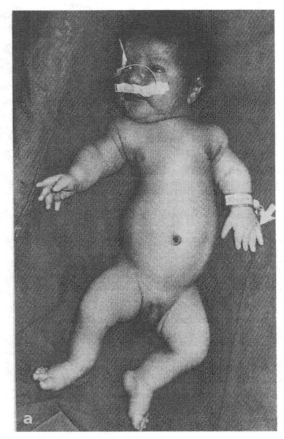

Fig. 6-1. (a) Newborn infant with contracted thorax. The polydactly of the hand (arrow) is partially obscured.

(b) Radiograph of pelvis and lower limbs. The tubular bones have bulbous ends but the pelvic configuration is indistinguishable from that of asphyxiating dysplasia.

(c) Chest radiograph showing a constricted thoracic cage and handlebar configuration of the high-situated clavicles. The heart is enlarged due to an associated cardiac defect

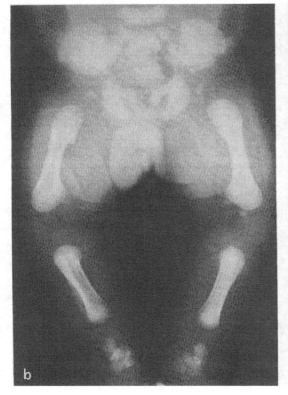

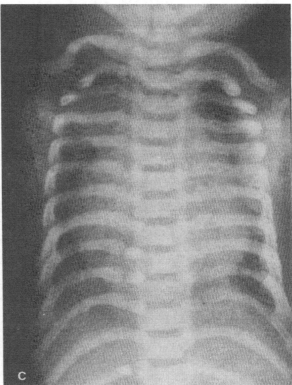

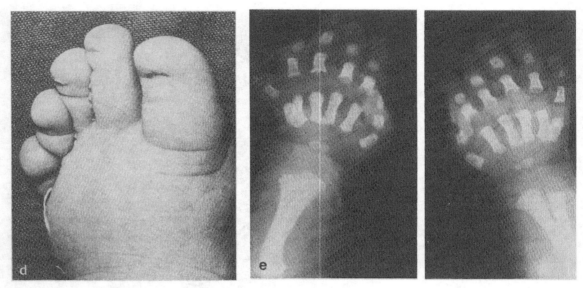

Fig. 6-1. (d) Underdevelopment of toenails.   (e) Hexadactyly and some underdevelopment of the phalanges

Chapter 7
Lethal Short Rib-Polydactyly Syndromes

Short rib-polydactyly syndromes in addition to asphyxiating thoracic dysplasia and chondroectodermal dysplasia have been recognized. SPRANGER et al. (1974) reviewed these conditions and defined the Saldino-Noonan and Majewski forms while NAUMOFF et al. (1977) reported a third variety. There is some overlap in these descriptions and delineation is not yet complete.

Short Rib-Polydactyly Syndrome Type I (Saldino—Noonan)

SALDINO and NOONAN (1972) described two stillborn siblings with severe thoracic dystrophy, gross micromelia, hypoplastic long bones, polydactyly, and multiple internal congenital abnormalities. The ribs were extremely short and the vertebral bodies were distorted with incomplete coronal clefts. The pelvis showed the small iliac bones with flattened acetabular roofs that are common to all the thoracic dystrophy syndromes. The femora were amorphous in appearance, with no corticomedullary demarcation and had the unusual characteristic of being pointed at both ends.

The changes in the limbs and vertebrae distinguish this condition from asphyxiating thoracic dysplasia and chondroectodermal dysplasia.

Short Rib-Polydactyly Syndrome Type II (Majewski)

MAJEWSKI et al. (1971) described a stillborn dwarf with severe rib reduction and polydactyly. The spine and pelvis were normal, but except for the tibiae the limb-shortening was not distinctive. Facial clefts and anomalies of the external ear were additional features. This disorder is extremely rare.

Short Rib-Polydactyly Syndrome Type III (Naumoff)

NAUMOFF et al. (1977) studied three dwarfed neonates and designated the condition short rib-polydactyly syndrome type III. These infants, two of whom were siblings, died from respiratory distress in the perinatal period. The disorder was characterized by marked shortening of the ribs, thoracic constriction, polydactyly, a short cranial base, bulging of the forehead, and flattening of the nasal bridge. Radiographically the vertebral bodies were underdeveloped and the tubular bones severely shortened with terminal spurs as in achondrogenesis. These latter changes were particularly obvious in the femora and tibiae. The iliac bones were small with flattened acetabular roofs and the pelvic changes were similar to those of achondroplasia.

Radiographically types I and III are very similar. The main difference in the tubular bones is that in type I the bones are very hypoplastic and may have pointed ends while in type III they are more well developed and bear lateral spurs.

Comment

The nosologic status of the short rib-polydactyly syndromes is somewhat uncertain. Indeed NAUMOFF et al. (1977) claimed that two of Spranger's Saldino-Noonan cases had features of type III rather than type I. The problem is compounded by the fact that type III closely resembles the achondrogenesis type II which was described by VERMA et al. (1975). Although the rare short rib-polydactyly syndrome type II is clearly a distinct entity, types I and III may simply represent varying degrees of chondro-osseous maturity in the same fundamental disorder. Indeed, as GORDON and BROWN (1976) pointed out in a case report of two affected premature infants, the pattern of skeletal ossification may be related to the stage of fetal development at which death occurs. This would have to occur very early if features such as marginal spiculation (Chap. 2, Fig. 2-3c) were to persist. On this basis these conditions could be etiologically homogeneous.

Although the relationship of the short rib-polydactyly syndrome is unclear, there have been several reports of affected siblings and parental consanguinity, and there is little doubt that inheritance is autosomal recessive in each instance. Antenatal diagnosis has been made (RICHARDSON et al., 1977) and should be used in at risk pregnancies. The clinical and radiographic features of the disorders in which marked thoracic dysplasia and polydactyly are components are summarized in Table 2.

Table 2. Disorders With Thoracic Dysplasia and Polydactyly

	Asphyxiating Thoracic Dysplasia (Jeune)	Chondroectodermal Dysplasia (Ellis-van Creveld)	Short rib-polydactyly syndrome Type I (Saldino-Noonan)	Short rib-polydactyly syndrome Type II (Majewski)	Short rib-syndrome type III (Naumoff)
Relative prevalence	Common	Uncommon	Common	Extremely rare	Rare
Clinical Features					
Thoracic constriction	++	+	+++	+++	+++
Polydactyly	+	++	++	++	++
Limb shortening	+	+	+++	+	++
Congenital heart disease	−	++	++	++	−
Other abnormalities	Renal disease	Ectodermal dysplasia	Genitourinary and gastrointestinal anomalies	Cleft lip and palate	Renal abnormalities
Radiographic features					
Tubular bone shortening	+	+	+++	++	+++
Distinctive features in femora	−	−	Pointed ends	−	Marginal spurs
Short, horizontal ribs	++	++	+++	+++	+++
Vertical shortening of ilia and flat acetabula	++	++	++	−	++
Defective ossification of vertebral bodies	−	−	++	−	+
Shortening of skull base	−	−	−	−	+

References

GORDON, I. R. S., BROWN, N. J.: The syndrome of micromelic dwarfism and multiple anomalies. Ann. Radiol. (Paris) **19**, 161 (1976).

MAJEWSKI, F., PFEIFFER, R. A., LENZ, W., MÜLLER, R., FEIL, G., SEILER, R.: Polysyndaktylie, verkürzte Gliedmaßen und Genitalfehlbildungen: Kennzeichen eines selbständigen Syndroms. Z. Kinderheilk. **111**, 118 (1971).

NAUMOFF, P., YOUNG, L. W., MAZER, J., AMORTEGUI, A. J.: Short Rib-Polydactyly Syndrome Type 3. Radiology **122**, 443 (1977).

References

Richardson, M. M., Beaudet, A. L., Wagner, M. L., Malini, S., Rosenberg, H. S., Lucci, J. A., Jr.: Prenatal diagnosis of recurrence of Saldino-Noonan dwarfism. J. Pediatr. **91**, 467 (1977).

Saldino, R. M., Noonan, C. D.: Severe thoracic dystrophy with striking micromelia, abnormal osseous development, including the spine, and multiple visceral abnormalities. Am. J. Roentgenol. **114**, 257 (1972).

Spranger, J., Grimm, B., Weller, M., Weissenbacher, G., Hermann, J., Gilbert, E., Krepler, R.: Short rib-polydactyly (SRP) syndromes, types Majewski and Saldino-Noonan. Z. Kinderheilk. **116**, 73 (1974).

Verma, I. C., Bhargava, S., Agarwal, S.: An autosomal recessive form of lethal chondrodystrophy with severe thoracic narrowing, rhizoacromelic type of micromelia, polydactyly and genital anomalies. Birth Defects **11**, 167 (1975).

40   Chapter 7 (Figs. 7-1a, b, c)

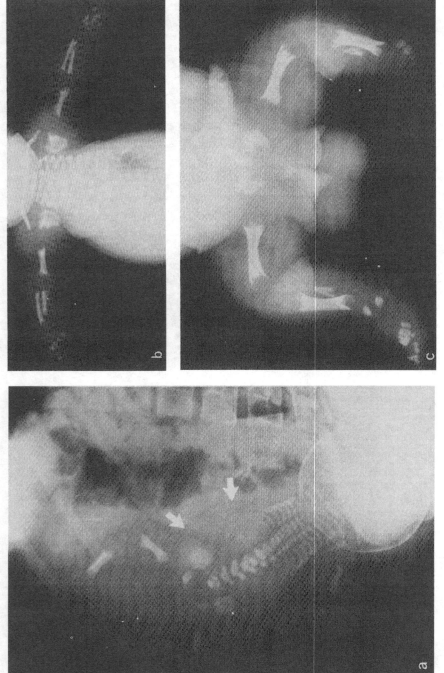

Case I

Fig. 7-1. (a) *In utero* radiograph. The constricted chest, small ilia, micromelia, and lateral spurs on the tubular bones are indicative of the short rib-polydactyly syndrome. The fat line around the prominent abdomen (*arrow*) indicates that fetal age is more than 32 weeks (b) Upper limbs are short, with lateral metaphyseal spicules, the scapulae are undercut, and thorax is severely constricted. (c) Lower limbs show a marked degree of lateral metaphyseal spiculation and small fibulae

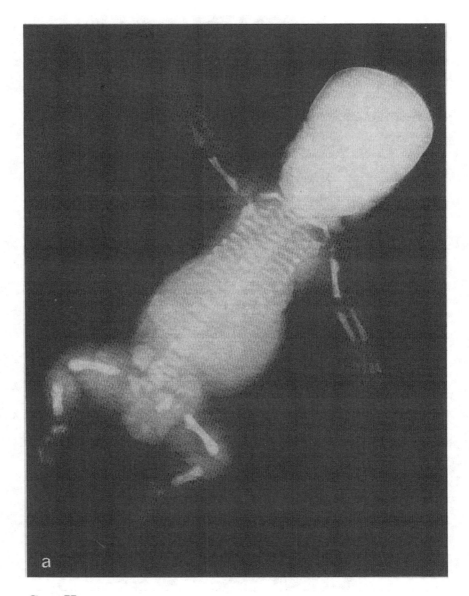

Case II

Fig. 7-2. (a) Whole-body radiograph of stillborn infant. Severe thoracic constriction is evident; pelvic and limb changes are seen to better advantage in 2. c, d)

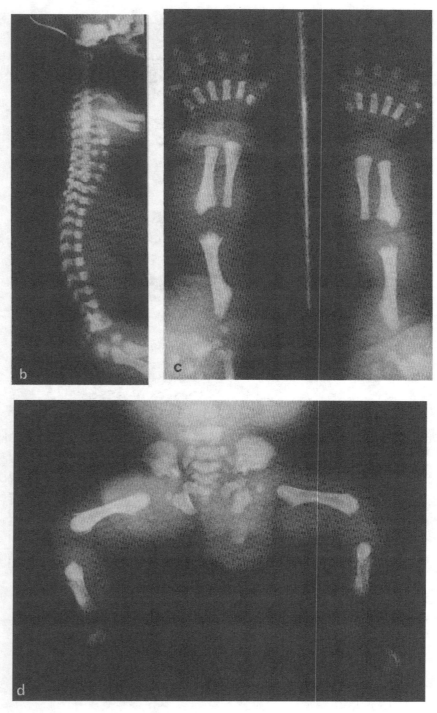

Case II

Fig. 7-2. (b) Severe rib-shortening and normal vertebrae. Length of the base of the skull is slightly reduced. (c) Upper limbs show micromelia, metaphyseal spurs in the humeri, and hexadactyly of the hands. (d) Pelvis has small iliac wings with irregularity of acetabular roof. Lateral metaphyseal spicules are evident in the femora and maturity of the capital femoral epiphyses is advanced

Chapter 7 (Figs. 7-3a, b)   43

Case III

Fig. 7-3. (a) AP chest of premature stillborn infant showing short ribs, thoracic constriction, high clavicles, and undercut lower margins of the scapulae

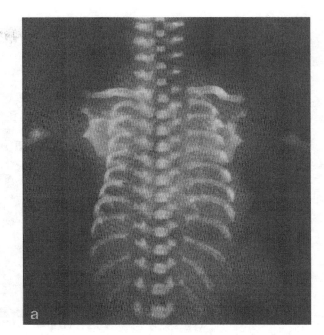

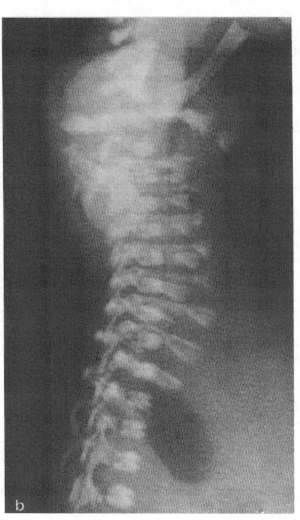

Fig. 7-3. (b) Lateral thoracic spine showing gross anteroposterior shortening of the ribs

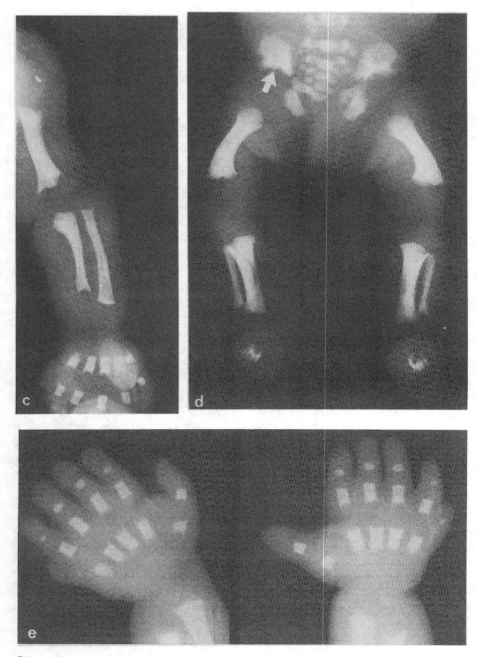

Case III

Fig. 7-3. (c) Micromelic upper limb; metaphyseal spiculation is not a feature in this case. (d) Pelvis shows a trident configuration of the acetabular roof (*arrow*). Lower limbs are shortened with some curvature of the femora. (e) Radiograph of the hands demonstrating polydactyly and lateral spiculation of short tubular bones

Comment

Radiographic differentiation of the various short rib-polydactyly syndrome can be difficult. Cases I and II fit into the Saldino-Noonan category but case III is atypical and cannot readily be classified (Naumoff type?)

Chapter 8
Chondrodysplasia Punctata

Chondrodysplasia punctata has a number of synonyms, including chondrodystrophia punctata, stippled epiphyses, chondrodystrophia calcificans congenita, and dysplasia epiphysealis punctata. The disorder is now conventionally subdivided into the potentially lethal rhizomelic autosomal recessive type and the more benign, autosomal dominant Conradi-Hünermann form (SPRANGER et al., 1971). An X-linked dominant variety of the latter has recently been reported and there is certainly residual heterogeneity. Chondrodysplasia punctata may also be classified in the following way:
1. Rhizomelic type—autosomal recessive
2. Conradi-Hünermann type—autosomal dominant and X-linked dominant forms
3. Other types
    Stippling of the epiphyses is also a feature of many other unrelated disorders, including:
        Multiple epiphyseal dysplasia
        Spondyloepiphyseal dysplasia
        Hypothyroidism
        Trisomy 18
        Trisomy 21
        Warfarin embryopathy
        Cerebrohepatorenal (Zellweger) syndrome
In all these conditions, as well as in the conventional forms of chondrodysplasia punctata, the stippling in the survivors disappears by the end of the second year of life.

1. Rhizomelic Type

Clinical Manifestations

Affected neonates have symmetric limb shortening which is maximal in the upper arms. The face is flat, with a depression of the nasal bridge and hypertelorism. Contractures of the limb joints may occur, while the fingers are stubby and fixed in flexion. Cataracts and ichthyosis are variable concomitants. Stillbirth or early death are usual, although a minority of patients survive beyond the first year. The long-term prognosis is poor.

Radiographic Features

The main radiographic changes are confined to limbs and spine.

I. Limbs. Rhizomelic shortening of the upper limbs predominates and involvement of the legs is variable. There is gross dysplasia of the metaphyses which is frequently most pronounced at the proximal ends of the long bones. These areas show extensive punctate calcific stippling in the form of multiple well-defined densities or larger highly irregular opacities which surround or occupy the ossification center.

II. Spine. Coronal clefts in lumbar and lower thoracic region are a noticeable feature. Stippling may occur but it is not always prominent.

Comment

The diagnosis may be suspected clinically, but radiographic studies are essential for diagnostic precision (GILBERT et al., 1976; HESELSON et al., 1977). As the condition is inherited as an autosomal recessive there is a 25% risk of recurrence. In view of the dismal prognosis and the genetic implications an accurate diagnosis is essential.

2. Conradi-Hünermann Type

Clinical Manifestations

The facies and dermal changes resemble those of the rhizomelic form of chondrodysplasia punctata. However the limb-shortening is less severe and is often symmetric. Structural abnormalities of the vertebral bodies are an additional feature which may cause spinal deformity. The stigmata and course are very variable; in severe forms early death may occur but in the milder cases survival is usual.

Radiographic Features

I. Limbs. In mild cases punctate calcification may be present only in the tarsus and carpus and in these patients there is no limb-shortening. In severe cases involvement is widespread and stippling may be seen in ankles, feet, patellae, hands, and wrists (pelvis, vertebrae, intervertebral discs, sternum, scapulae, rib cartilages, and mandible may also be involved). The stippled "paint spattered" changes may appear before ossification normally begins. Although the areas of endochondral ossification are predominantly affected the stippling may be periarticular and extend into the tissues outside the normal epiphyses.

II. Thorax and Pelvis. There are no special features apart from epiphyseal stippling.

III. Spine. Marked stippling in the vertebral and paravertebral regions is often a predominant feature.

IV. Other Areas. Calcification of the larynx and tracheal ring cartilage is sometimes found and KAUFMANN et al. (1976) have suggested that tracheal stenosis might be an important cause of mortality in these children. Chondrodysplasia punctata has been demonstrated radiographically in late pregnancy (HYNDMAN et al., 1976), but early antenatal diagnosis is not yet possible.

3. Other Types of Chondrodysplasia Punctata

The variability of the manifestations of the Conradi-Hünermann form probably reflects underlying heterogeneity. It is likely that there are a number of autosomal dominant types. SHEFFIELD et al. (1976) and HAPPLE et al. (1977) have proposed that there is an X-linked dominant variety which is lethal in males.

The radiographic abnormalities which permit differentiation of the rhizomelic and Conradi-Hünermann types are shown in Table 3.

Table 3

	Rhizomelic	Conradi-Hünerman
Tubular bones	Symmetric rhizomelic shortening of upper limbs with or without lower limb involvement. Metaphyses are grossly splayed and surrounded by stippling of variable degree	Shortening of limb bones is mild and asymmetric. Metaphyses not splayed. Stippling usually finely punctate
Thorax and Pelvis	No pathognomonic features	No pathognomonic features
Spine	Stippling usually absent or mild, coronal cleft on vertebral bodies invariably present	Vertebral and paravertebral stippling may be severe. Vertebral body anomalies and scoliosis may be present
Laryngeal and Tracheal Calcification	Not often present	Frequently present
Prognosis	Usually lethal	Frequently benign

References

GILBERT, E. F., OPITZ, J. M., SPRANGER, J. W., LANGER, L. O., WOLFSON, J. J., VISEKUL, C.: Chondrodysplasia punctata—rhizomelic form. Pathologic and radiologic studies of three infants. Eur. J. Pediatr. **123/2**, 89 (1976).

HAPPLE, R., MATTHIASS, H. H., MACHER, E.: Sex-linked chondrodysplasia punctata? Clin. Genet. **11**, 73 (1977).

HESELSON, N. G., CREMIN, B. J., BEIGHTON, P.: Lethal chondrodysplasia punctata. Clin. Radiol. in press (1978).

HYNDMAN, W. B., ALEXANDER, D. S., MACKIE, K. W.: Chondrodystrophia calcificans congenita. (The Conradi-Hünerman syndrome). Report of a case recognised antenatally. Clin. Pediatr. **15/4**, 311 (1976).

KAUFMANN, H. J., MAHBOUBI, S., SPACKMAN, T. J., CAPITANO, M. A., KIRKPATRICK, J.: Tracheal stenosis as a complication of chondrodysplasia punctata. Ann. Radiol. (Paris) **19/1**, 203 (1976).

SHEFFIELD, L. J., DANKS, D. M., MAYNE, V., HUTCHINSON, A. L.: Chondrodysplasia punctata—23 cases of a mild and relatively common variety. J. Pediatr. **89/6**, 916 (1976).

SPRANGER, J., OPITZ, J. M., BIDDER, U.: Heterogeneity of chondrodysplasia punctata. Humangenetik **11**, 190 (1971).

Chapter 8 (Figs. 8-1a, b)

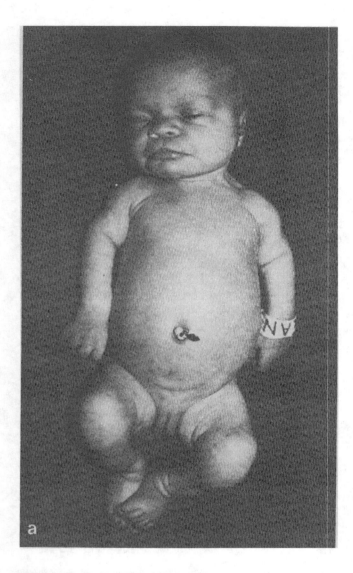

Case I

Fig. 8-1. (a) Affected infant who died three days after birth. Proximal (rhizomelic) limb shortening is very obvious

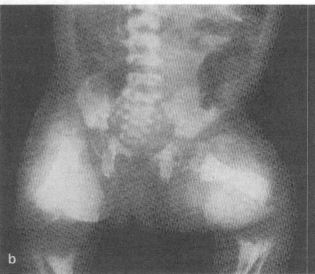

Fig. 8-1. (b) Pelvis and lower limbs showing rhizomelia. Stippling is present in pubis, sacrum, and femora

Chapter 8 (Figs. 8-1c, d)

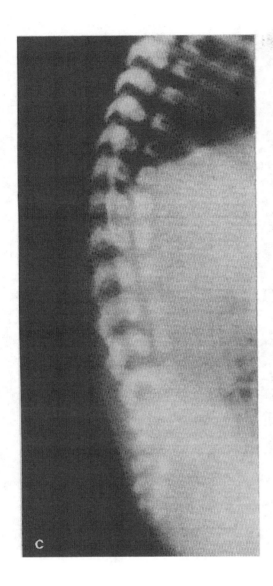

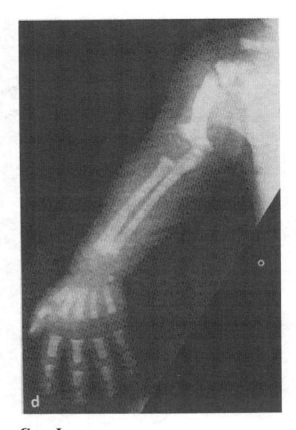

Case I

Fig. 8-1. (c) Coronal cleft vertebrae are a characteristic feature of the rhizomelic type of chondrodysplasia punctata

Fig. 8-1. (d) Upper limb showing severe rhizomelia and epiphyseal stippling

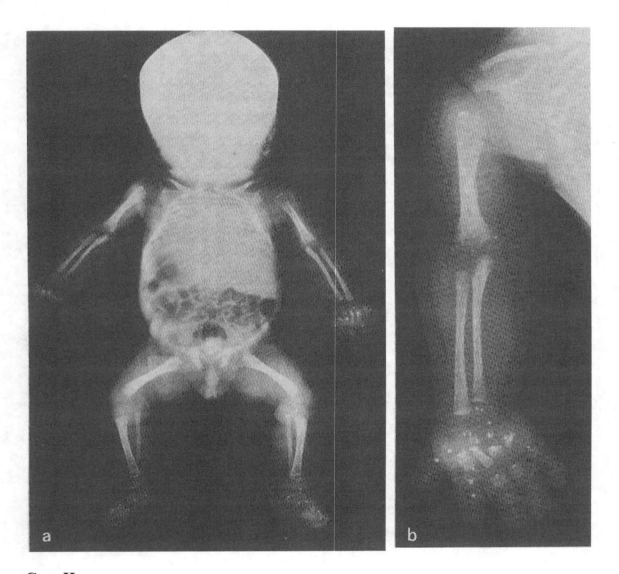

Case II

Fig. 8-2. (a) Newborn infant with the Conradi-Hünermann syndrome. Diffuse stippling with involvement of the spine is evident. (b) "Spattered paint" type of epiphyseal calcification with disturbed growth of the bones of the hand

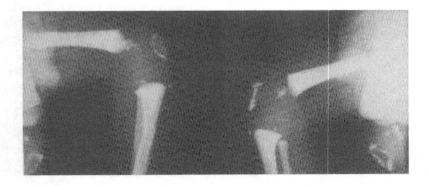

Case III

Fig. 8-3. Coarse calcification is seen around both knee joints of this infant

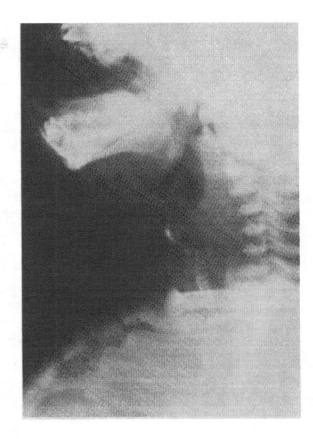

Case IV

Fig. 8-4. Calcification of the trachea in a 4-month-old infant. Stippling was also present in other epiphyseal centers

Chapter 9
Campomelic Dysplasia

There have now been more than 30 case reports of campomelic dysplasia. The disorder has been reviewed by several authors, including BECKER et al. (1975) and WEINER et al. (1976). The designation connotes "bent limbs," which are the most obvious clinical feature (MAROTEAUX et al., 1971).

Clinical Manifestations

The limbs are shortened to a mild degree with marked anterolateral bowing of the legs and talipes equinovarus. The face is flat, the ears low-set, and micrognathia with cleft palate is often present; hypoplasia of the tracheal rings has been reported (LEE et al., 1972). Death from respiratory insufficiency usually occurs in the neonatal period.

Radiographic Features

I. Limbs. The bowing of the femora is centered in the upper half of the bone while the angulation of the tibiae occurs in their lower half. The cortices of the bones are thinned at the convexity of the curve and the fibulae are hypoplastic.

II. Thorax and Pelvis. The chest is somewhat narrow with small scapulae, slender clavicles and gracile ribs.

III. Spine. The vertebrae show some platyspondyly and undermineralization. The bones of the pelvic girdle are a little underdeveloped.

IV. Skull. The vault is normal but the facial bones may be hypoplastic.

Comment

Campomelic dysplasia must be differentiated from hereditary tibial torsion and a number of syndromes in which congenital bowing of the long bones is a component (BLUMEL et al., 1957; NEWELL and DURBIN, 1976; THOMPSON et al., 1976). The etiology of campomelic dysplasia is uncertain, and there is controversy as to whether the condition is determined by genetic or environmental factors. Following a study of nine patients KHAJAVI et al. (1976) proposed that there were distinct "long limb" and "short limb" forms of campomelic dysplasia. The latter variety was further subdivided into craniosynostotic and normocephalic forms. The status of these disorders as separate entities is uncertain.

References

Becker, M. H., Feingold, M., Genieser, N. B.: Campomelic dwarfism. Birth Defects 11/6, 113 (1975).
Blumel, J., Eggers, G. W., Evans, E. B.: Eight cases of hereditary bilateral tibial torsion in four generations. J. Bone Joint Surg. 39 A, 1198 (1957).
Khajavi, A., Lachman, R. S., Rimoin, D. L., Shimke, R. N., Dorst, J. P., Ebbin, A. J., Handmaker, S., Perreault, G.: Heterogeneity in the campomelic syndromes: long and short bone varieties. Birth Defects 10/6, 93 (1976).
Lee, F. A., Isaacs, H., Strauss, J.: The "campomelic" syndrome. Am. J. Dis. Child. 124, 485 (1972).
Maroteaux, P., Spranger, J., Opitz, J. M., Kucera, J., Lowry, R. B., Schimke, R. N., Kagan, S. M.: Le syndrome campomélique. Presse Méd. 79, 1157 (1971).
Newell, R. L. M., Durbin, F. C.: The aetiology of congenital angulation of tubular bones with constriction of the medullary canal, and its relationship to congenital pseudoarthrosis. J. Bone Joint Surg. 58 B/4, 444 (1976).
Thompson, W., Oliphant, M., Grossman, H.: Bowed limbs in the neonate: significance and approach to diagnosis. Ann. Pediatr. (Paris) 5/1, 50 (1976).
Weiner, D. S., Benfield, G., Robinson, H.: Camptomelic dwarfism. Report of a case and review of the salient features. Clin. Orthop. 116, 29 (1976).

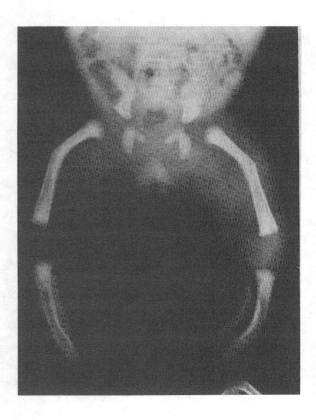

Fig. 9-1. Curvature of femora and tibia in affected neonate who died of respiratory distress. Iliac and pubic bones are underdeveloped

Chapter 10
Achondroplasia

Achondroplasia is by far the most common form of disproportionate dwarfism. Until recently the majority of newborn short-limbed dwarfs have been misdiagnosed as achondroplasts or achondroplasia variants and this has been the source of considerable confusion, both in the literature and in clinical practice (HARRIS and PATTON, 1971).

Clinical Manifestations

The newborn child with achondroplasia has rhizomelia, limb bowing, a bulky cranium, and a depressed nasal bridge. The buttocks are prominent due to lumbar lordosis and posterior angulation of the sacrum. The hand is stubby and lack of approximation of the digits gives a "trident" appearance. The prognosis for life and health in the perinatal period is reasonably good, but the large head can cause obstructed labor. Although the diagnosis can be reached on a clinical basis, radiographic studies are essential for confirmation. As with many other forms of skeletal dysplasia, the stigmata become increasingly obvious and specific with the passage of time. The clinical features of achondroplasia have been reviewed by SCOTT (1976).

Radiographic Features

I. Limbs. The tubular bones are short, thick, and often slightly curved. Their metaphyseal ends lack sharp margins of provisional calcification. The proximal ends of the femora are ill-defined and rounded, having an oval, lucent appearance from narrowing of the AP diameter; this is shown as a shelf in the lateral projection. In the legs the tibiae show some recession in the lateral view at the site of the anterior tubercle while the fibulae tend to be elongated. The epiphyseal centers at the knee are absent in the newborn. The upper limbs are rhizomelic, the upper humeri showing a lucent area similar to that seen in the femora. In the hands the middle and proximal phalanges are comparatively short and broad.

II. Thorax and Pelvis. Chest features are not notable though there may be some mild constriction of the thoracic cage.

The pelvis shows marked changes, the iliac wings being underdeveloped and squared off, with a "tombstone" configuration. The sacroiliac notch is narrow with a prominent medially directed spur and the acetabular roof is flat with a slightly irregular contour.

III. Spine. Progressive narrowing of the interpedicular distance in the AP projection is regarded as a hallmark of achondroplasia. This feature may not be present in the newborn, however, and its absence does not mitigate against the diagnosis. Indeed, interpediculate measurement with any degree of accuracy in this age group is difficult technically. The vertebral height is slightly diminished and the intervertebral disk spaces are widened. Anterior beaking or "bullet-nose" changes in the vertebrae may be evident on lateral views and mild kyphoscoliosis in the lumbar region may become apparent early in infancy.

IV. Skull. Defective growth occurs in all the bones which are preformed in cartilage. This results in a shortening of the skull base with narrowing of the foramen magnum, flattening of the nasal bridge, and prominence of the frontal region.

Comment

Radiological opinion may only be requested after some skeletal maturation has occurred. In young children the spine may show some wedging of individual vertebrae (particularly thoracolumbar), while the interpedicular narrowing of the lower canal becomes more evident. The femora lose their upper lucency with the development of the femoral necks and bony attachments such as the greater trochanter are exaggerated. The distal femoral metaphyses tend to become concave and partially envelop the metaphyses. The radiological features of achondroplasia in infancy and children have been reviewed in detail by LANGER et al. (1967) and SILVERMAN (1973).

About 80% of newborn achondroplasts represent new gene mutations and have normal parents. In these circumstances the diagnosis is not usually suspected antenatally. If one of the parents is an achondroplast and liable to transmit the gene, attempts at intrauterine diagnosis are worthwhile. This is only possible radiographically during the third trimester but in this way unforeseen complications at delivery may be forestalled. An unsuccessful attempt at antenatal diagnosis by radiography in early pregnancy has been reported by GLOBUS and HALL (1974).

In homozygous achondroplasia the infant receives an abnormal gene from each of a pair of achondroplast parents. This problem has been reviewed by HALL et al. (1969) and discussed in the context of thanatophoric dwarfism (see Chap. 4).

References

GLOBUS, M.S., HALL, B.D.: Failure to diagnose achondroplasia in utero. Lancet **1974/I**, 629.
HALL, J.G., DORST, J.P., TAYBI, H., LANGER, L.O., SCOTT, C.I., MCKUSICK, V.A.: Two probable cases of homozygosity for the achondroplasia gene. Birth Defects **5(4)**, 24 (1969).
HARRIS, R., PATTON, J.T.: Achondroplasia and thanatophoric dwarfism in the newborn. Clin. Genet. **2**, 61 (1971).
LANGER, L.O., JR., BAUMANN, P.A., GORLIN, R.J.: Achondroplasia. Am. J. Roentgenol. Radium Ther. Nucl. Med. **100**, 12 (1967).
SCOTT, C.I.: Achondroplastic and hypochondroplastic dwarfism. Clin. Orthop. **114**, 18 (1976).
SILVERMAN, F.N.: Achondroplasia: Intrinsic Diseases of Bone. Progress in Pediatric Radiology, Vol. IV, p. 94. Basel: Karger 1973.

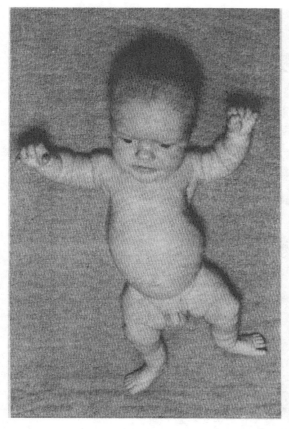 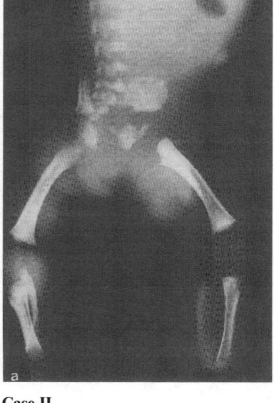

Case I

Fig. 10-1. Infant with achondroplasia. Proximal limb-shortening, depression of the nasal bridge, and a prominent forehead are the most obvious clinical features. (Courtesy of Dr. R. Harris, University of Manchester)

Case II

Fig. 10-2. (a) Oblique view showing a shelf in the upper femora and the configuration of the ilia from the side. The vertebral bodies have some degree of platyspondyly, which may be due to prematurity

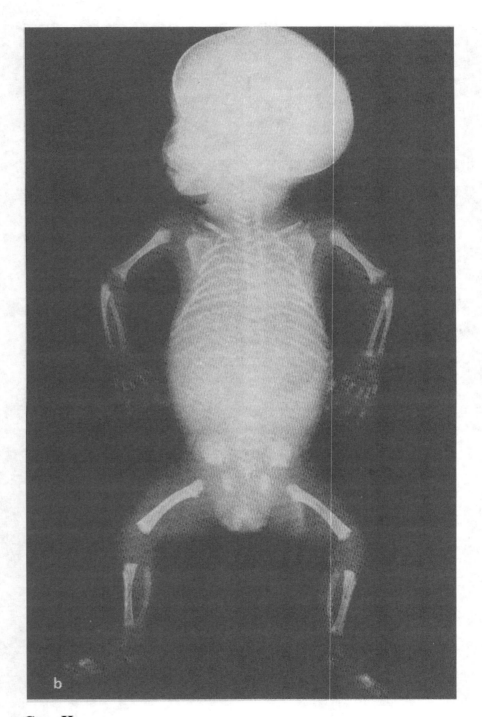

Case II

Fig. 10-2.(b) Whole-baby radiograph of a premature (32 week) stillborn achondroplast. The chest is bellshaped but ribs are comparatively normal. Iliac bones are square and the roof of the acetabulum is flat. Limb-shortening is not a prominent feature at this stage

Chapter 10 (Figs. 10-3a, b/10-4)

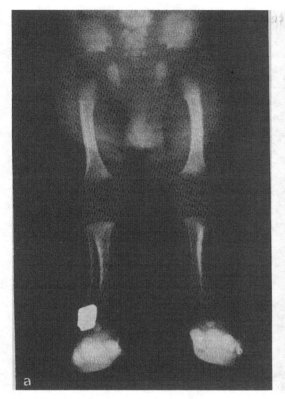 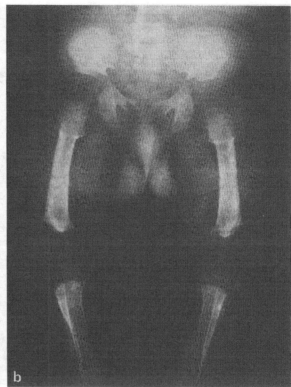

Case III

Fig. 10-3. (a) Full-term newborn achondroplast. The ilia have a square "tombstone" configuration, with a prominent medial spur. Upper femora are rounded and relatively lucent. These are distinctive and typical features. (b) At one month the changes in pelvis and upper limbs are more prominent, particularly the oval lucency of the upper femora

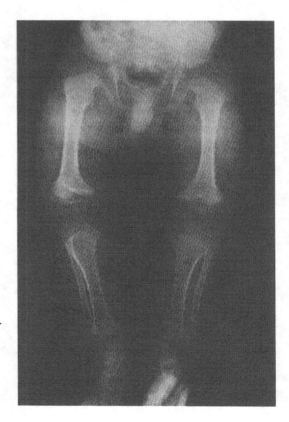

Case IV

Fig. 10-4. Appearance of pelvis and lower limbs in a 5-year-old achondroplast. Femoral heads are small and the femora are short, with prominent trochanters. Lower femoral metaphyses have a "chevron" configuration, due to invagination by the epiphyses

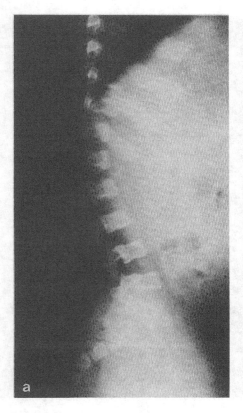
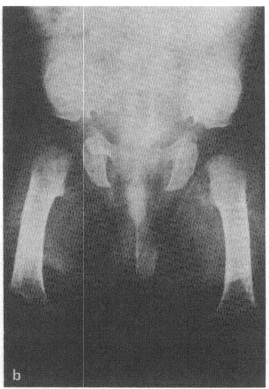
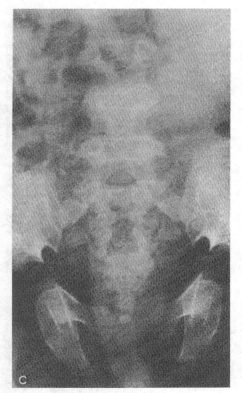

Case V

Fig. 10-5. (a) Lateral radiograph of the spine at one year showing short pedicles and increased intervertebral disk spaces. (b) Infant of 7 weeks. The square iliac bones, flat acetabular roofs, lucent upper femora, and absence of the femoral capital epiphyses are prominent features

Fig. 10-5. (c) The narrow interpediculate distances in the lower lumbar spine are seen in this coned view

Chapter 11
Diastrophic Dysplasia

This condition was first described by LAMY and MAROTEAUX (1960) when they reported three patients who had been originally diagnosed as atypical achondroplasia. The term "nanisme diastrophique", which was used by these authors, refers to the twisted habitus in this serious disorder. Diastrophic dysplasia is not uncommon and WALKER et al. (1972) were able to assemble a series of 51 cases.

Clinical Manifestations

The characteristics of the syndrome are short-limbed dwarfism, club feet, progressive scoliosis, and distinctive abnormalities of hands and ears. The thumb and great toe are displaced proximally and project at right angles in a "hitchhiker" position, while cystic degeneration distorts the pinna of the ear. The chronology of these changes is inconsistent, they may be present at birth or develop during infancy. Some joints are lax with dislocation or subluxation, while in others the range of movement is restricted. Cleft palate and micrognathia are present in a significant proportion of patients. The prognosis for life is reasonably good, although respiratory complications may be lethal in infancy. The stigmata, management, and prognosis in diastrophic dysplasia have been reviewed by HOLLISTER and LACHMAN (1976).

Radiographic Features

I. Limbs. Dislocations of joints and flexion deformities are important features and severe, rigid club feet are a consistent finding. The long tubular bones are shortened and broadened to a variable degree and there is delay in the appearance of the epiphyseal centers, which may be flattened. The hands show some ulnar deviation and the first metacarpal has a characteristic progressive abduction deformity. This metacarpal may be shortened and triangular or ovoid in shape and the other bones in the hand and foot are frequently truncated and unevenly ossified.

II. Thorax and Pelvis. There are no special features in the thorax. The pelvis not infrequently shows hip dysplasia, the poorly formed acetabula being associated with dislocation.

III. Spine. In severely affected patients thoracolumbar scoliosis appears at or soon after birth. The scoliosis is progressive and may be accompanied by slight platyspondyly. Hypoplasia of the bodies of the cervical vertebrae is common and subluxation may occur, particularly at C1–C2.

Comment

Diastrophic dysplasia is inherited as an autosomal recessive and parents who have produced an affected child are, therefore, at a one in four recurrence risk for any subsequent pregnancy. The condition can be recognized *in utero* during the third trimester by standard radiographic techniques, but as yet early antenatal diagnosis has not been achieved.

In mild cases the radiographic appearance may not be impressive in the neonate. The problems of radiographic diagnosis in early infancy have been discussed by LANGER (1965), CREMIN and JARRET (1970), KOZLOWSKI and BARYLAK (1974), and SAULE (1975).

In the neonatal period the combination of the shortness of the limbs, dislocations, and club feet may suggest this diagnosis. The distinctive digital changes and ear distortion may be present at this time but they are not usually prominent early features. The club feet and rigid joints may lead to confusion with arthrogryposis multiplex congenita but the dwarfism, good muscle mass, and osseous abnormalities in diastrophic dysplasia readily permit differentiation.

References

CREMIN, B. J., JARRET, J.: Diastrophic dwarfism. Aust. Radiol. **14**, 84 (1970).
HOLLISTER, D. W., LACHMAN, R. S.: Diastrophic dwarfism. Clin. Orthop. **114**, 61 (1976).
KOZLOWSKI, K., BARYLAK, A.: Diastrophic dwarfism. Aust. Radiol. **18**, 398 (1974).
LAMY, M., MAROTEAUX, P.: Le nanisme diastrophique. Presse Méd. **68**, 1977 (1960).
LANGER, L. O.: Diastrophic dwarfism in early infancy. Am. J. Roentgenol. **93**, 399 (1965).
SAULE, H.: Diastrophic Dwarfism. Radiology **15/2**, 50 (1975).
WALKER, B. A., SCOTT, C. I., HALL, J. G., MURDOCH, J. L., MCKUSICK, V.: Diastrophic dwarfism. Medicine **51**, 41 (1972).

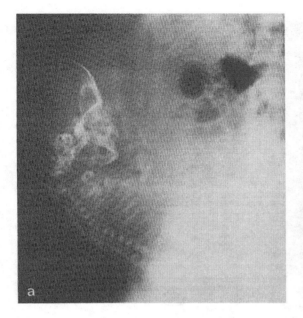
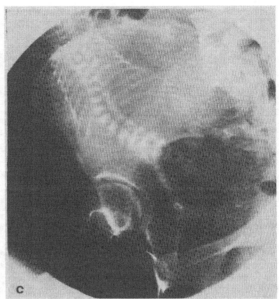
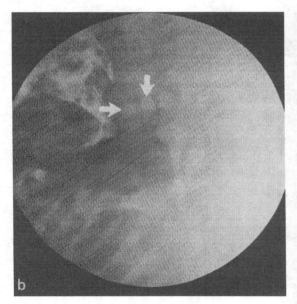
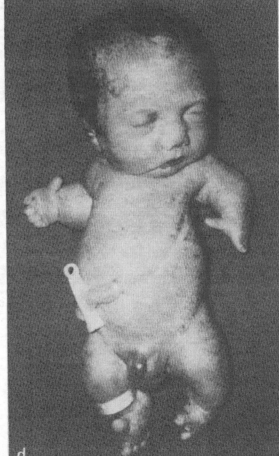

Case I

Fig. 11-1. (a) *In utero* lateral radiograph showing micromelia, twisting of the spine, and some contraction of the thoracic cage. (b) *In utero* localized close-up view of the upper limb showing the extended "hitchhiker" (*arrows*) deformity of thumb. (c) *In utero* oblique radiograph demonstrating the narrow thoracic cage and twisted spine (the relative gap between bodies and pedicles seen in lower spine is due to the projection). (d) Stillborn infant. Micromelia, distortion of the limbs, and the hitchhiker deformity of the thumbs and big toes are clearly seen

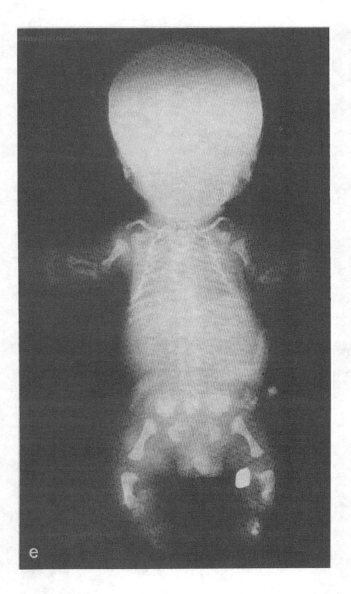
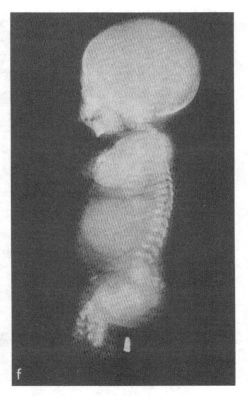
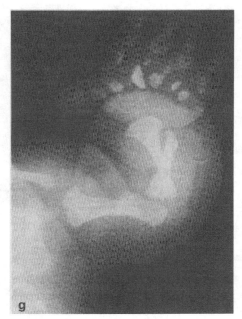

Case I

Fig. 11-1. (e) AP whole body radiograph showing spinal curvature and micromelia; the hips are subluxed. (f) lateral radiograph showing marked shortening of the limbs with some metaphyseal flaring. (g) Short upper limb, fixed abduction of the thumb (hitchhiker deformity) and maldevelopment of hand bones. The changes in this neonate are unusually severe and hitchhiker thumbs are not invariably present in infancy

Chapter 11 (Figs. 11-2a, b, c)

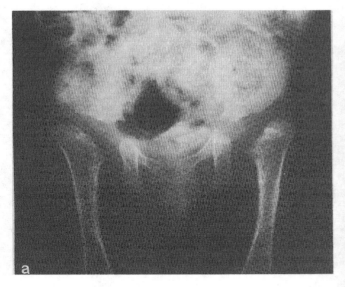

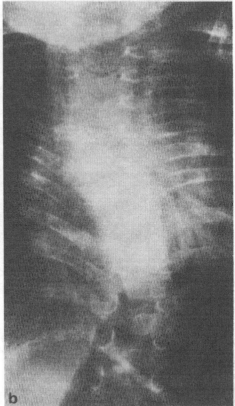

Case II

Fig. 11-2. (a) Pelvis of a 5-month-old infant showing defective ossification of the acetabular roofs and bilateral hip dislocation. (b) Thoracic spine showing scoliosis in its lower half.

Fig. 11-2. (c) Upper limb showing shortening and dislocation of the proximal end of the radius. Although the typical thumb abnormality had not yet appeared, the joint dislocations, deformity of the ear pinnae, and clubbed feet were prominent features

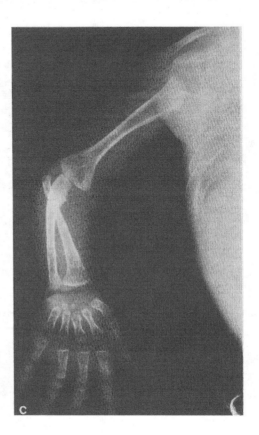

Chapter 12
Metatropic Dysplasia

This rare disorder was delineated by Maroteaux et al. (1966). "Metatropic" refers to the changing bodily proportions which are the result of progressive spinal malalignment and shortening of the trunk relative to the limbs. Case reports can be recognized in the early literature under the redundant title "hyperplastic achondroplasia". There are different varieties of this condition, including a rare, severe form which is lethal in the neonate.

Clinical Manifestations

In the newborn the thorax is narrow, the trunk normal in length, and the limbs short (Larose and Gay, 1969; Jenkins et al., 1970). Cleft palate may be present and the large joints are prominent and rigid, though the finger joints may be hyperextensible. A tail-like appendage attached to the coccyx is an inconsistent but important aid to diagnosis. Progressive kyphoscoliosis develops during early childhood and the affected adult is severely deformed.

Radiographic Features

I. Limbs. The limb bones are short with characteristic trumphet-like flaring of their metaphyses. The appearance of ossification centers may be delayed. With growth, the proximal ends of the femora develop a "battle-axe" configuration,

II. Thorax and Pelvis. The thoracic cage is narrowed, with short ribs and a prominent sternum. In the pelvis the iliac wings are small but flared, the acetabular roofs are horizontal and irregular, and the pubic bones are ill-developed.

III. Spine. In the spine there is severe generalized platyspondyly, with gross widening of the disk spaces and defective mineralization of the lower lumbar vertebrae. In later childhood the vertebrae become wedge-shaped with humped-up central and dorsal portions. Progressive spinal malalignment and secondary distortion of the thorax occurs.

Comment

Rimoin et al. (1976) and Kozlowski et al. (1976) have emphasized that there are a number of incompletely defined variants of metatropic dysplasia. Pseudometatropic dysplasia, in which joint laxity leads to spinal deformity and reversal of bodily proportions, falls into this category (Bailey, 1971).

The Kniest syndrome has also been classified with metatropic dysplasia, although it is now accepted that it is a separate entity. Following the original report by KNIEST (1952), a series of eight patients have been described by SIGGERS et al. (1974). Affected neonates have short limbs and stiff joints, while cleft palate, inguinal hernia, and clubfeet may also be present. Progressive kyphoscoliosis leads to trunk shortening during childhood, and myopia, retinal detachment and deafness are potentially serious hazards. At birth radiographs of the skeleton show undermineralization, platyspondyly, and irregular expansion of epiphyses and metaphyses of long bones. These changes are much less marked than those occurring in metatropic dysplasia.

Micromelia with a flared metaphyseal "dumbbell" configuration may also be seen in the Weissenbacher-Zweymuller syndrome. This chondrodysplasia is characterized by micrognathia and coronal cleft vertebrae rather than platyspondyly (HALLER et al., 1975; CORTINA et al., 1977).

References

BAILEY, J. A.: Forms of dwarfism recognisable at birth. Clin. Orthop. **76**, 150 (1971).
CORTINA, H., APARICI, R., BELTRAN, J., ALBERTO, C.: The Weissenbacher-Zweymuller syndrome. Pediatr. Radiol. **6**, 109 (1977).
HALLER, J. O., BERDON, W. E., ROBINOW, M., SLOVIS, T. L., BAKER, D. H., JOHNSON, G. F.: The Weissenbacher-Zweymuller syndrome of micrognathia and rhizomelic chondrodysplaia at birth with subsequent normal growth. Am. J. Roentgenol. **125**, 936 (1975).
JENKINS, P., SMITH, M. B., McKINNEL, J. S.: Metatropic dwarfism. Br. J. Radiol. **43**, 561 (1970).
KNIEST, W.: Zur Abgrenzung der Dysostosis enchondralis von der Chondrodystrophie. Z. Kinderheilk. **70**, 633 (1952).
KOZLOWSKI, K., MORRIS, L., REINWEIN, H., SPRAGUE, P., TAMAELA, L. A.: Metatropic dwarfism and its variants (report of six cases). Aust. Radiol. **20**, 367 (1976).
LAROSE, J. H., GAY, B. G.: Metatropic dwarfism. Am. J. Roentgenol. **106**, 156 (1969).
MAROTEAUX, P., SPRANGER, J., WIEDEMANN, H. R.: Der metatropische Zwergwuchs. Arch. Kinderheilk. **173**, 211 (1966).
RIMOIN, D. L., SIGGERS, D. C., LACHMAN, R. S., SILBERBERG, R.: Metatropic dwarfism, the Kniest syndrome and pseudoachondroplastic dysplasias. Clin. Orthop. **114**, 70 (1976).
SIGGERS, D., RIMOIN, D., DORST, J., DOTY, S., WILLIAMS, B., HOLLISTER, D., SILBERBERG, R., CRANLEY, R., KAUFMAN, R., McKUSICK, V.: The Kniest syndrome. Birth Defects **10/9**, 193 (1974).

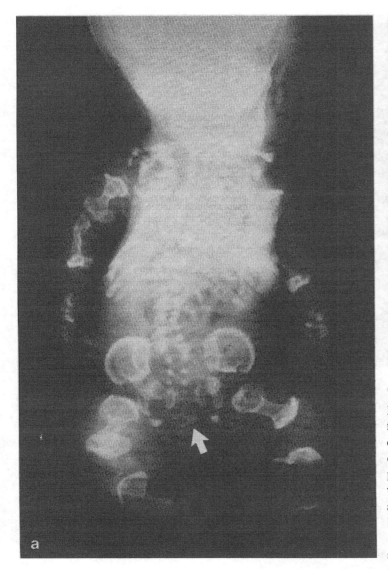
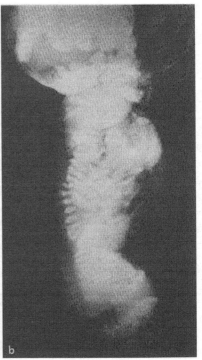

Case I

Fig. 12-1. (a) AP radiograph of an infant who died from severe respiratory distress soon after birth. The features of this lethal form of the condition are platyspondyly, marked micromelia with widely expanded metaphyses and an ossified tail (*arrow*). (Courtesy of Dr. G. Perri, Pisa). (b) Lateral radiograph demonstrating severe platyspondyly and shortness of the ribs. (Courtesy of Dr. G. Perri, Pisa)

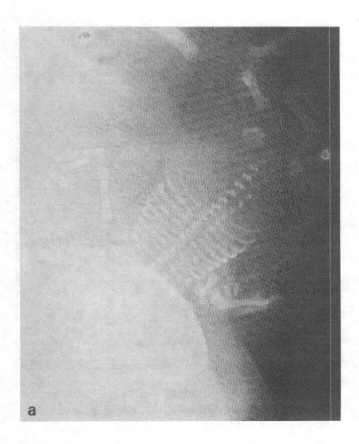

Case II

Fig. 12-2. (a) The mother of this infant was radiographed for hydramnios at 35 weeks. The short limbs and small iliac bones of the fetus were noted and a diagnosis of an indeterminate skeletal dysplasia was made. A Cesarian section was performed a week later and the infant died shortly after delivery. (b) Pelvis and limbs, demonstrating small iliac bones with a trident appearance of the acetabular roofs and metaphyseal flaring of the femora. The fibulae are disproportionately long

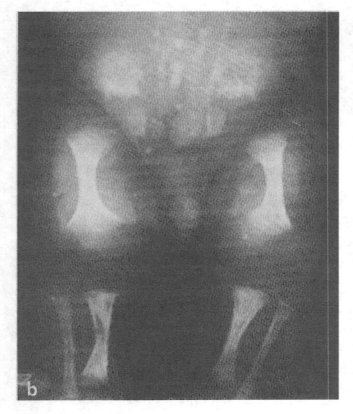

Comment

These two cases illustrate some of the difficulties in diagnosing metatropic dwarfism.
1. Both cases showed micromelia, metaphyseal flaring, and spinal underdevelopment, but early death prevented us from knowing if the characteristic changes would have developed.
2. Case II could also be classified as some form of yet undefined spondylometaepiphyseal dysplasia.

Chapter 13
Spondyloepiphyseal Dysplasia Congenita

The spondyloepiphyseal dysplasias are a heterogeneous group of disorders in which abnormalities in the epiphyses and spine predominate. As the stigmata may be present at birth or appear in later childhood, the condition is conventionally classified into "congenita" and "tarda" types. The features of the congenita form have been discussed in detail by SPRANGER and WIEDEMANN (1966).

Clinical Manifestations

Affected neonates have short limbs and a flat face. Cleft palate and talipes equinovarus are often present, the hips may be dislocated, and the elbow joints cannot be fully extended. The prospects for survival are good, but spinal malalignment and a barrel chest are evident in early childhood and severe dwarfing ultimately ensues. Myopia and retinal detachment are potentially serious late complications.

Radiographic Features

I. Limbs. Limb changes are not prominent although the femoral heads and necks tend to be dysplastic and the epiphyses at the knee and calcaneum appear late.

II. Thorax and Pelvis. The thorax is bell-shaped in the frontal projection, the iliac wings are somewhat flared, with relatively broad bases, and the pubic bones are underossified.

III. Spine. The diagnostic features are ovoid or pear-shaped vertebral bodies. Irregular ossification results in severe platyspondyly. Hypoplasia of the odontoid process of C2 is often present.

Comment

In the neonate the radiological characteristics may not be striking but changes soon become apparent in the spine, pelvis and femoral heads. With further development the spinal abnormalities become increasingly prominent while the iliac wings and pubis remain underdeveloped. The radiological features have been reviewed by KOZLOWSKI et al. (1968) and SPRANGER and LANGER (1970).

The term "Morquio syndrome" is often used for any syndrome of dwarfism and spinal malalignment, including the spondyloepiphyseal dysplasias. In the strict sense, however, this eponym should be reserved for a specific condition, mucopolysaccharidosis type IV, which is not recognizable at birth.

Spondyloepiphyseal dysplasia congenita is inherited as an autosomal dominant. Atypical cases are not uncommon, and there is little doubt that there is at least one autosomal recessive variety. Other variants have also been reported, such as a lethal form in which metaphyseal changes, hydrocephalus and occipital encephalocoele are additional features (DINNO et al., 1976).

References

DINNO, N. D., SHEARER, L., WEISSKOPF, B.: Chondrodysplastic dwarfism, cleft palate and micrognathia in a neonate, a new syndrome? Eur. J. Pediatr. **123/1**, 39 (1976).
KOZLOWSKI, K., BUDZINSKA, A.: Spondylo-epiphyseal dysplasia congenita. Ann. Radiol. (Paris) **11**, 367 (1968).
SPRANGER, J. W., LANGER, L. O.: Spondyloepiphyseal dysplasia congenita. Radiology **94**, 313 (1970).
SPRANGER, J., WIEDEMANN, H. R.: Dysplasia spondyloepiphysaria congenita. Helv. Pediat. Acta. **21**, 598 (1966).

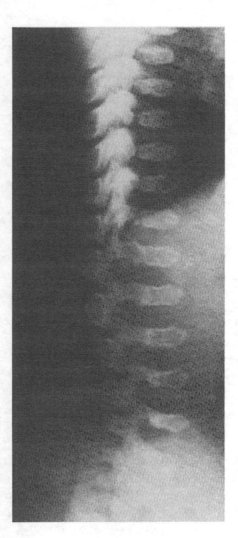

Fig. 13-1. Lateral spine of an affected neonate showing severe flattening of vertebral bodies. At this stage of development there are no other diagnostic radiographic features

Chapter 14
Mesomelic Dysplasia

The term "mesomelic" implies limb-shortening which is maximal in the forearms and lower legs and this feature predominates in a number of rare disorders which are recognisable in the neonate. The best known of these bear the eponyms "Nievergelt," "Langer," "Robinow," "Rheinardt," and "Werner," but several other less clearly defined entities exist. The clinical, radiological, and genetic implications of the mesomelic dysplasias have been reviewed by SILVERMAN (1973) and KAITILA et al. (1976).

These conditions are all compatible with survival and good general health. With the exception of the Langer form, which probably represents the homozygous state of dyschondrosteosis, (ESPIRITU et al., 1975) they are all inherited as autosomal dominants. Their manifestations, other than mesomelia and dwarfism are shown in Table 4.

Table 4

Syndrome	Clinical Features	Radiographic Features	References
Nievergelt	Flexion deformities	Rhomboidal tibia	YOUNG and WOOD (1975)
Langer	Mandibular hypoplasia	Madelung deformity	LANGER (1967)
Robinow (fetal face syndrome)	Abnormal facies and genitals	Hemivertebrae and rib fusions	ROYINOW et al. (1969) GIEDION et al. (1975)
Reinhardt	Limb-bowing	Synostosis in the carpus and tarsus	REINHARDT and PFEIFFER (1967), REINHARDT (1976)
Werner	Polydactyly and absence of thumbs	Gross tibial hypoplasia	PASHAYAN et al. (1971)

Comment

Several of the mesomelic dysplasias are confined to a single family and can, therefore, be regarded as "private syndromes." Doubtless others await delineation. Antenatal recognition has not been reported.

In acromelic dysplasia shortening of the tubular bones of the hands and feet constitutes an additional feature (MAROTEAUX et al., 1971). The main radiographic features are a Madelung deformity of the forearms, hypoplasia of the tibia, and peripheral dysostosis. This disorder is inherited as an autosomal recessive (BEIGHTON, 1974).

Peripheral dysostosis, in which cone-shaped epiphyses and premature closure of the growth plate result in digital shortening, may occur in isolation or as a component of a number of syndromes. The term "acrodysostosis" is applied to peripheral dysostosis in association with nasal hypoplasia and mental retardation (ROBINOW et al., 1971).

References

BEIGHTON, P.: Autosomal recessive inheritance in the mesomelic dwarfism of Campailla and Martinelli. Clin. Genet. **5**, 363 (1974).

ESPIRITU, C., CHEN, H., WOOLEY, P. V.: Mesomelic dwarfism as the homozygous expression of dyschondrosteosis. Am. J. Dis. Child. **129**, 375 (1975).

GIEDION, A., MATTAGLIA, G. F., BELLINI, F., FANCONE, G.: The radiological diagnosis of the fetal face (Robinow) syndrome (mesomelic dwarfism and small genitalia). Report of three cases. Helv. Paediatr. Acta **30/4—5**, 409 (1975).

KAITILA, I. I., LEISII, J. T., RIMOIN, D. L.: Mesomelic skeletal dysplasia. Clin. Orthop. **114**, 94 (1976).

LANGER, L. O.: Mesomelic dwarfism of the hypoplastic ulna, fibula, and mandibular type. Radiology **89**, 654 (1967).

MAROTEAUX, P., MARTINELLI, B., CAMPAILLA, E.: Le nanisme acromesomelique. Presse Méd. **79**, 1839 (1971).

Pashayan, H., Fraser, F. C., McIntyre, J. M., Dunbar, J. S.: Bilateral aplasia of the tibia, polydactyly and absent thumb in father and daughter. J. Bone Joint Surg. **53 B**, 495 (1971).

REINHARDT, K.: A dominant-autosomal transmitted micromelia with dysplasia of radius and ulna (Reinhardt-Pfeiffer syndrome). V. International Congress of Human Genetics, Mexico, D.F. 1976.

REINHARDT, K., PFEIFFER, R. A.: Ulna-fibulare Dysplasie. Eine autosomal-dominant vererbte Mikromesomelie ähnlich dem Nievergeltsyndrom. Fortschr. Geb. Röntgenstr. Nuklearmed. **107**, 379 (1967).

ROBINOW, M., PFEIFFER, R. A., GORLIN, R. J., MCKUSICK, V. A., RENUART, A. W., JOHNSON, G. F., SUMMITT, R. L.: Acrodysostosis: A syndrome of peripheral dysostosis, nasal hypoplasia, and mental retardation. Am. J. Dis. Child. **121**, 195 (1971).

ROBINOW, M., SILVERMAN, F. N., SMITH, H. D.: A newly recognised dwarfing syndrome. Am. J. Dis. Child. **117**, 645 (1969).

SILVERMAN, F. N.: Progress in Pediatric Radiology. Intrinsic Diseases of Bones, Vol. IV, p. 546. Basel: Karger 1973.

YOUNG, L. W., WOOD, B. P.: Nievergelt syndrome (mesomelic dwarfism type Nievergelt). Birth Defects **11/5**, 81 (1975).

Chapter 14 (Figs. 14-1a, b, c)

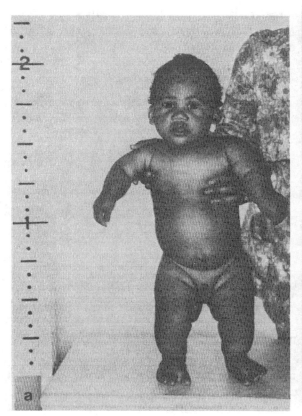
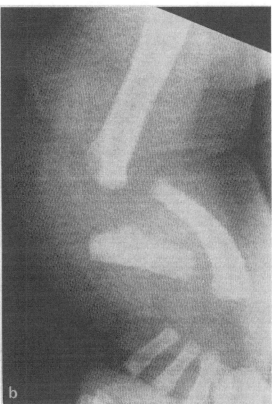

Case I

Fig. 14-1. (a) Infant with mesomelic dysplasia. Limb shortening is maximal in the forearms and lower legs. (b) Marked shortening and curvature of radius and ulna

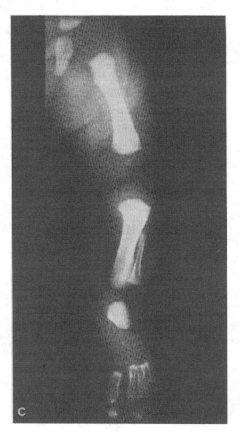

Fig. 14-1. (c) Shortening is particularly evident in the fibula

Case II

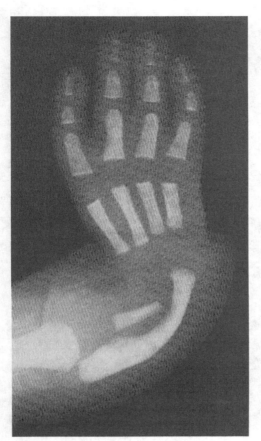

Fig. 14-2. Newborn infant with hypoplastic radius and an absent thumb. This infant presented with a visceral defect and deformity of a single limb

Comment

Case II is beyond the scope of this book, but it is included to illustrate a point of differential diagnosis. Bone abnormalities of this type may be associated with thrombocytopaenia or vertebral, anal, cardiac, tracheal, esophageal, and renal anomalies.

Chapter 14 (Figs. 14-3a, b, c)

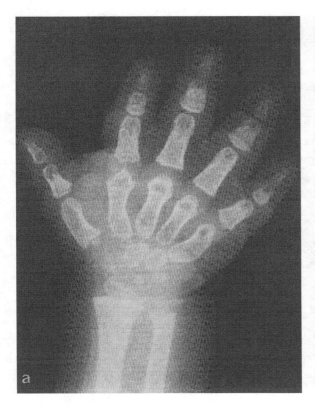
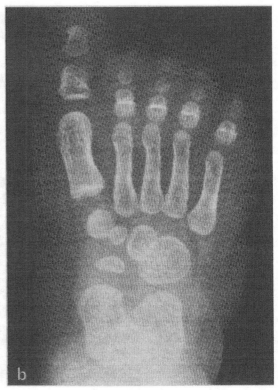

Case III

Fig. 14-3. (a and b) Case of acrodysostosis. No mesomelia was present in this 14-month-old female who has peripheral dysostosis with shortening of hand and foot bones and advanced maturation of carpal and tarsal bones. (c) Skull showed hypertelorism and some brachycephaly. In this lateral view the characteristic features of nasal hypoplasia and a large mandibular angle are shown

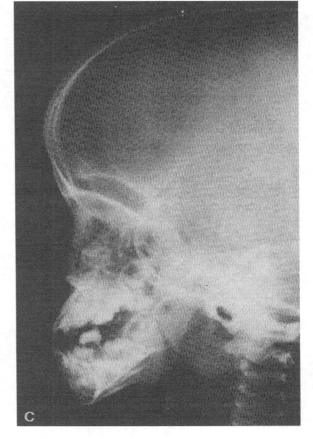

Comment

Case III could well be included in a separate section but is presented here as an introduction to a complex subject. At a later stage cone-shaped epiphyses will develop at the proximal ends of the phalanges.

Chapter 15
Larsen Syndrome

Since the first case descriptions by LARSEN et al. (1950), more than 50 cases have been recognized. It is probable that there are distinct autosomal dominant and recessive forms of the condition, but these have not yet been clearly delineated (MAROTEAUX, 1975). The course and management have been discussed by HABERMANN et al. (1976), OKI et al. (1976), and MICHEL et al. (1976).

Clinical Manifestations

Articular hypermobility is the predominant feature and the affected neonate may present as a "floppy infant." The knee joints are especially lax and genu recurvatum is often gross. Dislocation of the hip joints and talipes equinovarus may occur. The radial heads are frequently dislocated, and consequently the elbows have a paradoxical limitation of full extension and rotation. Structural vertebral anomalies and ligamentous laxity predispose to spinal malalignment, which is variable in degree. The nasal bridge is wide and depressed, producing a characteristic "dish face." The terminal phalanges, particularly those of the thumb, are widened into a spatulate configuration. Cardiac malformations are an inconsistent feature and the prognosis for life and health is dependent upon the presence or absence of cardiorespiratory embarrassment and spinal cord compression.

Radiographic Features

At birth the radiographic changes are essentially the result of joint laxity. Dislocation of the radial heads and the hips may be demonstrated, while subluxation or an undue range of movement may be evident at other sites. In some affected infants hemivertebrae are present in the upper spine. A supernumerary ossification center in the calcaneum is pathognomonic for the Larsen syndrome; this is not usually seen before the end of the first year. At a later stage extra ossicles sometimes develop in the carpus.

The radiographic changes in the Larsen syndrome have been reviewed by KOZLOWSKI et al. (1974).

Comment

The Larsen syndrome is probably much more common than is generally recognized. The diagnosis can be made on a clinical basis but radiographic studies are of confirmatory value.

Accumulating evidence indicates that the autosomal dominant form is comparatively benign, while the autosomal recessive type is potentially lethal. As yet neither variety has been recognized *in utero*.

References

Habermann, E. T., Sterling, A., Dennis, R. I.: Larsen syndrome: a heritable disorder. J. Bone Joint Surg. **58**/4, 558 (1976).
Kozlowski, K., Robertson, F., Middleton, R.: Radiographic findings in Larsen's syndrome. Aust. Radiol. **18**/3, 336 (1974).
Larsen, L. J., Schottstaedt, E. R., Bost, F. D.: Multiple congenital dislocations associated with a characteristic facial abnormality. J. Paediatr. **37**, 574 (1950).
Maroteaux, P.: Heterogeneity of Larsen's syndrome. Arch. Fr. Pediatr. **32**/7, 597 (1975).
Michel, L. J., Hall, J. E., Watts, H. G.: Spinal instability in Larsen's syndrome: report of three cases. J. Bone Joint Surg. **58**/4, 562 (1976).
Oki, T., Terashima, Y., Murachi, S., Nogami, H.: Clinical features and treatment of joint dislocations in Larsen's syndrome. Report of three cases in one family. Clin. Orthop. **119**, 206 (1976).

Chapter 15 (Figs. 15-1/15-2a, b, c)

Case I

Fig. 15-1. Infant with characteristic scooped-out face due to wide depression of the nasal bridge

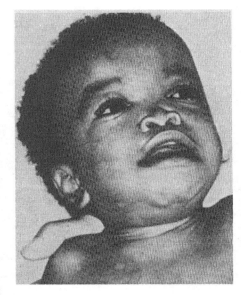

Case II

Fig. 15-2. (a) Lateral skull radiograph showing hypoplasia of the nasal and facial bones. (b) Lateral view of the foot showing a typical additional anterior ossification center in the calcaneum (*arrow*). (c) Radiograph of the hand and arm 3-year-old child. The superior radio-ulnar joint is dislocated and the metacarpo-phalangeal joint of the fifth finger is subluxed. Supernumerary ossicles are present in the carpus

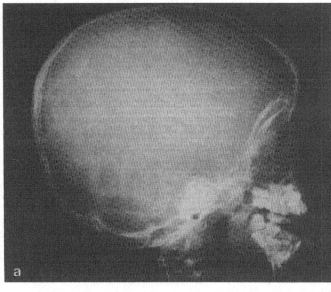

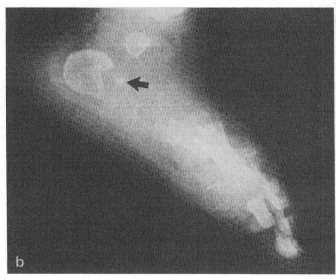

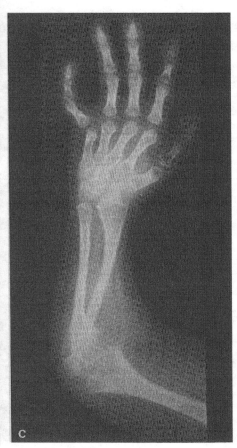

Chapter 16
Cleido-Cranial Dysplasia

Cleidocranial dysplasia is a benign condition in which varying degrees of clavicular maldevelopment are associated with characteristic changes in the skull. The disorder is unlikely to be suspected in a neonate unless a positive family history has prompted radiographic studies.

Clinical Manifestations

Individuals with cleidocranial dysplasia resemble one another, having a small triangular face and a bulky brow. Clavicular hypoplasia may permit undue mobility of the shoulder girdle but affected infants are otherwise normal. Adult height is somewhat reduced, but apart from dental problems and a wide variant of uncommon inconsistent concomitants, cleidocranial dysplasia is comparatively harmless.

Radiographic Features

I. Limbs. Shortness of the limbs is not usually notable but a generalized delay in ossification of the tubular bones with some mild degree of stunting of stature is not unusual. In later childhood supernumerary epiphyses, particularly of the second and fifth metacarpals, are common while cone-shaped epiphyses of the phalanges are a nonspecific feature (GIEDION, 1967).

II. Thorax and Pelvis. Clavicular dysplasia may not be a prominent radiographic feature. Complete absence occurs in only 10% of patients (SOULE, 1946) and more often small, lateral or medial stumps are present. A bony defect between the two segments of the clavicle may simulate a pseudoarthrosis. Narrowing of the thorax may occasionally provoke some mild respiratory distress. Supernumerary ribs are frequently present and the sternum may be incompletely ossified.

Delayed ossification of the central portion of the pubic bones is an important diagnostic sign in infants and only ischial and iliac bones may be visible in the pelvic brim.

III. Spine. The normal biconvex infant vertebral bodies tend to persist into early childhood. Inconsistent spinal anomalies may result from lack of vertebral maturation.

IV. Skull. The predominant skull changes are multiple wormian bones and wide sutures. The wormian bones form a mosaic in the posterior portion of the skull. In the neonate the skull shows some demineralization and with growth there may be basilar invagination. The anterior fontanelle remains open and tends to advance forward, while the vault becomes brachycephalic, with an increased biparietal diameter. The facial bones are generally underdeveloped and dental anomalies are common. The deciduous dentition may be relatively normal, although sometimes delayed.

Comment

The predominant radiological features of this condition are the result of failure of midline growth; thus skull and pelvic abnormalities are the most consistent while other changes, including those of the clavicles, are variable.

Cleidocranial dysplasia is inherited as an autosomal dominant. The considerable variation of expression which may be encountered within any particular kindred has been emphasized by FORLAND (1962), FAURE and MAROTEAUX (1973), and JARVIS and KEATS (1974). Affected individuals often remain unrecognized, and the disorder usually constitutes little more than a harmless curiosity (JACKSON, 1951).

References

COLE, W.R., LEVIN, S.: Cleidocranial dysostosis. Br. J. Radiol. **24**, 549 (1951).
FAURE, C., MAROTEAUX, P.: Progress in Pediatric Radiology. Intrinsic Diseases of Bones. Cleidocranial Dysplasia, Vol. IV, p. 211. Basel: Karger 1973.
FORLAND, M.: Cleidocranial dysostosis. Am. Med. **33**, 792 (1962).
GIEDION, A.: Cone-shaped epiphyses of the hands and their diagnostic value. The tricho-rhino-phalangeal syndrome. Ann. Radiol. (Paris) **10**, 322 (1967).
JACKSON, W.P.U.: Osteo-dental dysplasia (cleido-cranial dysostosis) the "Arnold head." Acta Med. Scand. **139**, 292 (1951).
JARVIS, L.J., KEATS, T.E.: Cleidocranial dysostosis, a review of 40 new cases. Am. J. Roentgenol. Radium Ther. Nucl. Med. **121**, 5 (1974).
SOULE, A.B.: Mutational dysostosis (cleidocranial dysostosis). J. Bone Joint Surg. **28**, 81 (1946).

Chapter 16 (Figs. 16-1a, b)

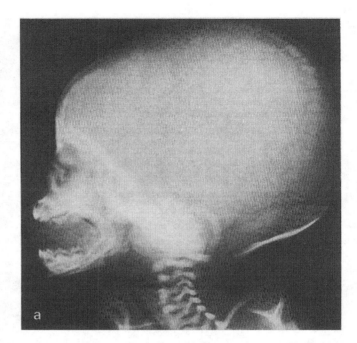

Case I

Fig. 16-1. (a) One-month-old child with multiple wormian bones in the calvarium

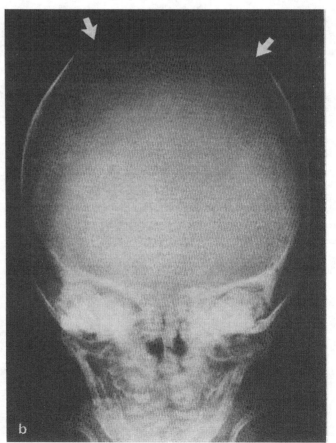

Fig. 16-1. (b) AP projection. Anterior fontanelle is widely open (*arrows*)

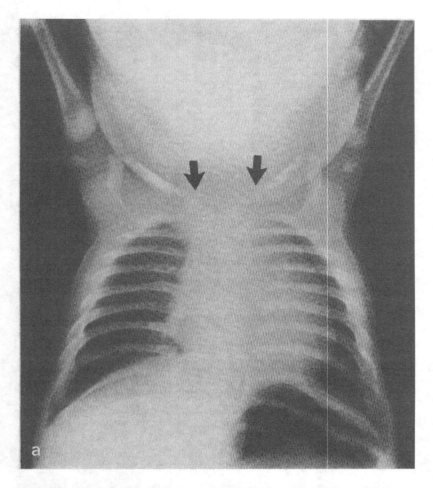

Case II

Fig. 16-2. (a) Chest of a 9-month-old infant showing mild hypoplasia of medial ends of clavicles (*arrows*). The thoracic cage is slightly small and the thymusheart configuration is normal

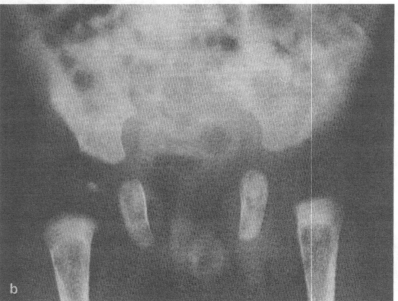

Fig. 16-2. (b) Pelvis, showing the highly characteristic absence of the central portion of the pubic bones

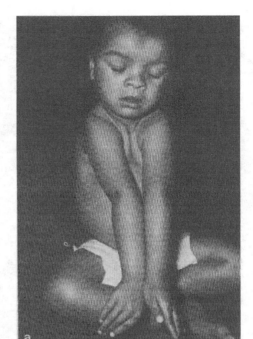

Case III

Fig. 16-3. (a) Five-year-old child demonstrating the typical abnormal mobility of the shoulders and arms, due to deficiency of the clavicles

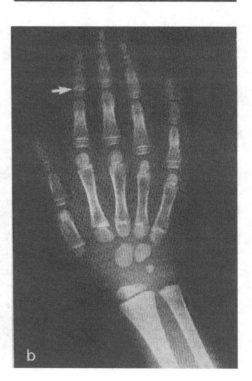

Fig. 16-3. (b) Supernumerary ossification conters at the bases of the second and fifth metacarpals. The one-shaped epiphysis (*arrow*) is a frequent but nonspecific finding

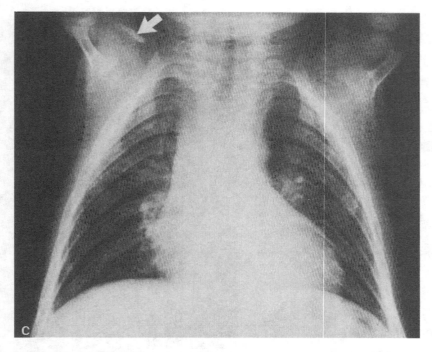

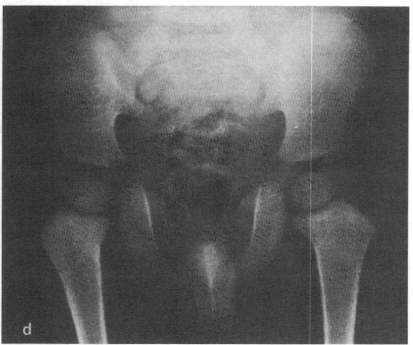

Case III

Fig. 16-3. (c) The clavicle is absent on the left side while only a rudimentary portion is present on the right (*arrow*).

Fig. 16-3. (d) Characteristic absence of the central portion of the pubic bones

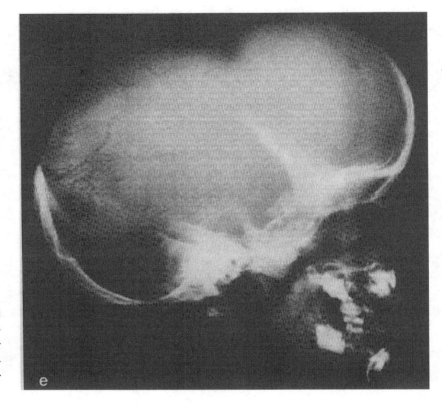

Case III

Fig. 16-3. (e) Lateral skull radiograph showing multiple wormian bones, basilar invagination, and deficiency of the vault and anterior fontanelle

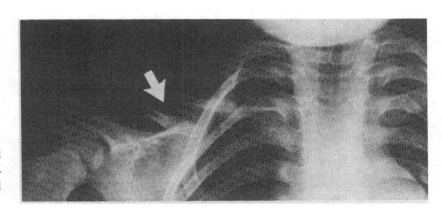

Case IV

Fig. 16-4. Six-year-old child with a pseudoarthrosis (*arrow*) in a poorly developed clavicle

Chapter 17
Osteogenesis Imperfecta Congenita

Osteogenesis imperfecta is one of the most common genetic skeletal dysplasias. The condition is conventionally classified into the congenita form, where the marked changes are present at birth, and the tarda variety, in which bone fragility only becomes evident in later childhood. The eponyms "Vrolik" and "Porak-Durante" are sometimes applied to the former type, and "Lobstein" and "Van de Hoeve" to the latter. It must be emphasized that although osteogenesis imperfecta is certainly heterogeneous, the congenita and tarda forms do not necessarily represent separate genetic entities.

Clinical Manifestations

Infants with osteogenesis imperfecta congenita may sustain multiple fractures *in utero* or during delivery, and limb deformity consequent upon these events may be evident at birth. The calvarium may be poorly ossified, forming a soft caput membranaceum, and in this situation fatal intracranial bleeding is not unusual. Blueness of the sclera and widening of the bitemporal diameter are other inconsistent clinical features. The majority of neonates are less severely affected and survival is not unusual (CURRARINO and BROOKSALER, 1973; CHONT, 1941; KING and BOBECHKO, 1971). The frequency of fractures is very variable but they are sometimes associated with marked soft tissue swelling, increased local heat, and tenderness due to hypercallosis.

Radiographic Features

I. Limbs. The tubular bones of the lower limbs are generally the most severely involved. These bones are frequently bowed, bulky and irregular and may appear collapsed upon themselves in a "piano accordion" fashion. Varying degrees of osteoporosis are present and sometimes a honeycomb cystic appearance may be seen. Multiple fractures are frequent and abundant callus is a prominent radiographic feature. Many affected infants will have less florid changes. In these children the tubular bones are slender and gracile with thin cortices except where angulation and fracture cause cortical thickening.

II. Thorax and Pelvis. Chest changes include irregularity of ribs, which are often beaded in appearance, and multiple fractures, particularly in the upper thoracic cage. Lack of ossification in severe cases may make the pelvis almost rudimentary.

III. Spine. In the severely affected neonate platyspondyly may be present. In the young child the porotic process may lead to wedged or biconcave "fish" vertebrae.

IV. Skull. In the skull the vault may be affected to such a degree that it is not visible in intrauterine radiographs. In cases with less marked demineralization a mosaic of wormian bones is an outstanding feature. The invariable presence of multiple wormian bones is most helpful in diagnosis.

Demineralization is prominent in the severe potentially lethal congenita form of osteogenesis imperfecta. The tarda form is much more common and although it may be diagnosed in infancy, pathologic fractures usually draw attention to the condition between the age of two and three.

Comment

Osteogenesis imperfecta is usually inherited as an autosomal dominant, although rare autosomal recessive forms certainly exist (HORAN and BEIGHTON, 1975). The basic defect is unknown and precise delineation has not yet been achieved.

From the practical point of view, the sporadic infant with severe or lethal osteogenesis imperfecta congenita poses a difficult problem as it is often impossible to give a meaningful assessment of recurrence risks. It must be emphasized that the "thick bone" and "thin bone" classification, as described by FAIRBANK (1951) is purely a radiological concept and is unhelpful from the genetic point of view. The condition can be recognized *in utero* during the third trimester (HELLER et al., 1975; NAVANI and SARZIN, 1967), but as with many other lethal bone dysplasias, early antenatal diagnosis is not yet possible. Nevertheless, late diagnosis is important, as Cesarian section will minimise risk of fractures and intracranial bleeding during delivery.

References

CHONT, L. K.: Osteogenesis imperfecta. Report of twelve cases. Am. J. Roentgenol. **45**, 850 (1941).
CURRARINO, G., BROOKSALER, F.: Progress in Pediatric Radiology. Intrinsic Diseases of Bones. Osteogenesis Imperfecta, Vol. IV, p. 346. Basel: Karger 1973.
FAIRBANK, H. A. T.: An Atlas of General Affections of the Skeleton, 1st Ed. Edinburgh: Livingstone 1951.
HELLER, R. R., WINN, K. J., HELLER, R. M.: The prenatal diagnosis of osteogenesis imperfecta congenita. Am. J. Obstet. Gynaecol. **121/4**, 572 (1975).
HORAN, F., BEIGHTON, P.: Autosomal recessive inheritance of osteogenesis imperfecta. Clin. Genet. **8/2**, 107 (1975).
KING, J. D., BOBECHKO, W. P.: Osteogenesis imperfecta. An orthopaedic description and surgical review. J. Bone Joint Surg. **53B**, 72 (1971).
NAVANI, S. V., SARZIN, B.: Intra-uterine osteogenesis imperfecta. Review of the literature and a report of the radiological and necropsy findings in 2 cases. Br. J. Radiol. **40**, 449 (1967).

Chapter 17 (Figs. 17-1/17-2)

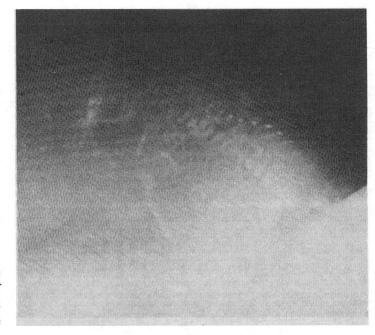

Case I

Fig. 17-1. *In utero* radiograph. The vault is unossified so that only base of skull and jaws are visible. The thin ribs and upper limb bones show multiple fractures

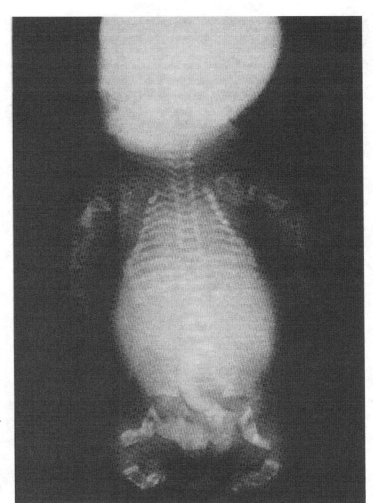

Case II

Fig. 17-2. Whole-body radiograph of stillborn infant. Deficient calvarial ossification, fractured "beaded" ribs, platyspondyly, small ilia, and typical "piano accordion" fractured limbs are evident

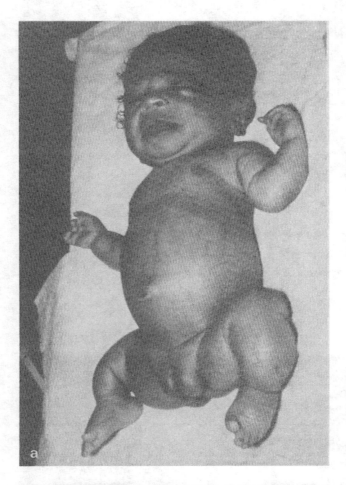

Case III

Fig. 17-3. (a) Three-week-old infant with bent, swollen legs due to multiple fractures. A clinical diagnosis was made before radiographs were taken

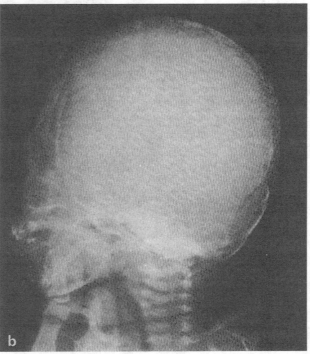

Fig. 17-3. (b) Multiple wormian bones and deossification of the vault of the skull

Chapter 17 (Fig. 17-3c)

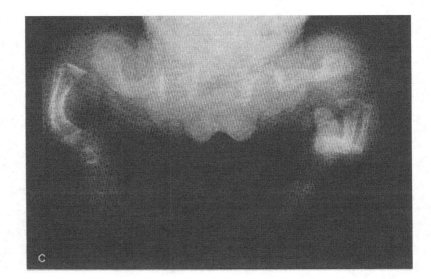

Case III

Fig. 17-3. (c) Lower limbs showing porotic deformed bones with thin cortices

Chapter 18
Hypophosphatasia

Hypophosphatasia, a rare condition which was delineated by RATHBUN (1948), is conventionally classified according to age of onset, and "infantile," "juvenile," and "adult" forms are recognized (CURRARINO, 1973). Often these subdivisions may be indistinct (JAMES and MOULE, 1966). Alternately, the disorder is divided into congenita, tarda, and latent varieties. This separation may be artificial, as MACPHERSON et al. (1972) have identified mild and severe forms within the same kindred. Nevertheless, the congenita form is often lethal and hypophosphatasia warrants consideration in this context.

Clinical Manifestations

The calvarium may be poorly ossified in the neonate and thus the contents of the cranium are vulnerable to bleeding and contusion. Stillbirth is frequent and respiratory distress in early infancy is not unusual. The limbs may be short and deformed by multiple fractures, and the clinical picture may resemble osteogenesis imperfecta congenita. The serum concentration of alkaline phosphatase is consistently low while the urinary excretion of phosphoethanolamine is elevated. The conditions can be differentiated, therefore, on this basis.

The neonatal cases are frequently lethal but in the less severely affected individual survival is possible. Skeletal fragility persists throughout childhood, and bowing of the tubular bones, stunting of stature, and dental problems commonly occur.

Radiographic Features

I. Limbs. In the neonatal form there is deficient ossification of the whole skeleton although the changes in tubular bones are variable in severity. There may be gross nonossification so that only the coarse and ragged central portions of the bones are apparent. More commonly the long bones have metaphyseal porosis in which there is a streaky, irregular, and spotty ossification. These coarsely ossified areas become widened and frayed and produce a bizarre rachitic appearance which is pathognomonic at this age. Intrauterine rubella may give "celery-stick" streaking of the metaphyses and congenital syphilis may produce metaphyseal lucent bands but combined deossified skull and limb lesions are only seen in hypophosphatasia.

II. Thorax and Pelvis. These regions are underossified in severe forms.

III. Spine. The vertebral bodies are flat and poorly formed in severe cases.

IV. Other Features. The skull may be globular and boneless, the calvarium being represented by a caput membranaceum. Cranial abnormalities vary from partial ossification, with the parietal bones appearing to float in an overtranslucent vault, to a generalized porosis with wide open sutures.

In less severely affected infants the changes are less striking and the condition may attract attention because of the widened cranial sutures, the lack of metaphyseal mineralisation or the angulations and fractures in the tubular bones. In survivors beyond the first year of life premature closure of the cranial sutures may result in craniostenosis.

Comment

Although hypophosphatasia is rare, Kozlowski et al. (1976) were able to assemble data concerning 24 cases from nine pediatric centers. Of these, three had the neonatal lethal type of the condition and 18 the severe infantile form. Inheritance is autosomal recessive and the heterozygous carrier of the gene can be recognized by the presence of minor clinical and biochemical abnormalities (Rubecz et al., 1974).

Antenatal radiographic diagnosis has been reported (Currarino et al., 1957). More recently lack of cranial ossification in an infant at risk has been demonstrated at the sixteenth week of pregnancy by ultrasonography (Rudd et al., 1976).

References

Currarino, G.: Progress in Pediatric Radiology. Intrinsic Diseases of Bones. Hypophosphatasia, Vol. IV, p. 469. Basel: Karger 1973.
Currarino, G., Neuhauser, E. B. D., Reyersbach, G. C., Sobel, E. H.: Hypophosphatasia. Am. J. Roentgenol. 78, 392 (1957).
James, W., Moule, B.: Hypophosphatasia. Clin. Radiol. 17, 368 (1966).
Kozlowski, K., Sutcliffe, J., Barylak, A., Harrington, G., Kemperdick, H., Nolte, K.: Hypophosphatasia—a review of 24 cases. Pediatr. Radiol. 5, 103 (1976).
MacPherson, R. I., Krocker, M., Houston, C. S.: Hypophosphatasia. J. Assoc. Can. Radiol. 23, 16 (1972).
Rathbun, J. C.: "Hypophosphatasia." A new developmental anomaly. Am. J. Dis. Child. 75, 822 (1948).
Rubecz, I., Mehes, K., Klujber, L., Bozzay, L., Weisenbach, J., Fenyvasi, J.: Hypophosphatasia: screening and family investigation. Clin. Genet. 6, 155 (1974).
Rudd, N. L., Miskin, M., Hoar, D. I., Benzie, R., Doran, T. A.: Prenatal diagnosis of hypophosphatasia. N. Engl. J. Med. 295, 146 (1976).

Chapter 18 (Figs. 18-1/18-2a, b)

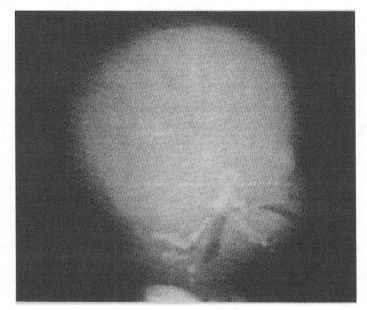

Case I

Fig. 18-1. Complete absence of ossification of the calvarium giving a "boneless" skull appearance in a lethal case

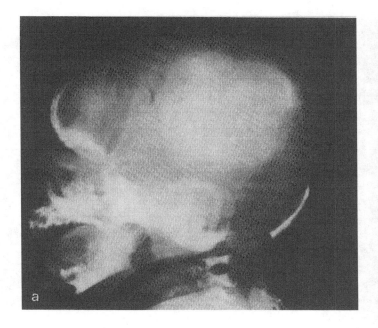
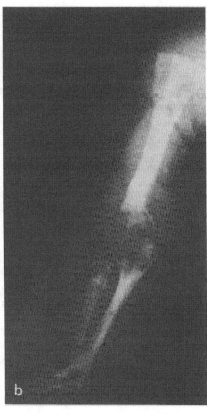

Case II

Fig. 18-2. (a) Foor ossification of the calvarium; the parietal bones appear to float in the skull vault. (b) Upper limb showing altered bone texture, with sclerotic and lucent areas and grossly frayed metaphyses

Chapter 19
Osteopetrosis and Other Sclerosing Bone Dysplasias

Increased bone density, with or without abnormal modeling, is a feature of a number of uncommon disorders of the neonate. The "precocious" or "malignant" form of osteopetrosis is the best known of these, but pycnodysostosis and sclerosteosis can also be recognized in early infancy. The designations "Albers-Schönberg" disease and "marble bones" are often used loosely and incorrectly for conditions of this type. In the strict sense, Albers-Schönberg disease is the benign or delayed autosomal dominant form of osteopetrosis, which is not usually recognizable in the neonate. The manifestations of this group of disorders have been reviewed by BEIGHTON et al. (1977).

The usual mode of presentation of the precocious form of osteopetrosis is anemia and failure to thrive. Hepatosplenomegaly and a progressive blood dyscrasia develop and in the later stages compression of cranial nerves and pathologic fractures may occur. The majority of infants with the disorder succumb to overwhelming infection before the end of the first year. The features of this autosomal recessive condition have been discussed in detail by SLY et al. (1972) and LORIA CORTES et al. (1977).

Radiographic Features

The predominant feature of osteopetrosis is generalized skeletal sclerosis.

I. Limbs. Increased density is characteristic, but there is also abnormal modeling of the metaphyses with diminished marrow space in the shafts of the tubular bones. In early infancy, however, these changes are very variable and periosteal layering may also feature. The bones are brittle and the sequelae of pathologic fractures may be evident. In the growing skeleton an endobone or "bone within bone" appearance is seen. Horizontal stratifications are present in the metaphyses of the long tubular bones and failure of modelling in these regions produces a flask-shaped configuration. In the short tubular bones of the extremities, lack of modelling is not prominent but metaphyseal sclerosis and central endobone formation is very evident.

II. Thorax and Pelvis. Dense bone may not be a feature until after infancy. During the growing period the iliac wings may show convex and radiating striations.

III. Spine. The vertebral end plates are sclerotic and endobone formation is common.

IV. Skull. Sclerosis initially involves the basal bones, later the calvarium is involved and vertical "hair on end" striae may develop. The facial bones are usually relatively spared.

Comment

The radiographic changes are age related and in the early stages accurate diagnosis is not always an easy matter. Indeed, failure to recognize the condition radiographically *in utero* has been reported (GOLBUS et al., 1976). Other conditions enter into the differential diagnosis and normal physiologic growth sclerosis may be a source of confusion. Disturbance of metaphyseal growth is indicated by alternating bands of lucency rather than density and these may be seen in prematurity, meconium ileus, and congenital syphilis (CREMIN and FISHER, 1970). In infancy hypervitaminoses and cortical hyperostosis, which also cause abnormal sclerosis, can be recognized by their different clinical presentation.

Prenatal recognition of osteopetrosis was reported by JENKINSON et al. (1943). However, although the skeleton in this case was diffusely dense, some doubt has been cast on the diagnosis (GRAHAM et al., 1973).

Generalized skeletal sclerosis, without defective modelling, occurs in pycnodysostosis (MAROTEAUX and LAMY, 1962). In this autosomal recessive disorder, the coronal sutures are wide, the angle of the mandible is obtuse, and the terminal phalanges are hypoplastic. Although the bones are fragile, hematologic problems do not arise and the prognosis for general health is good.

Sclerosteosis is a rare condition in which partial or total syndactyly of the second and third digits is associated with progressive skeletal overgrowth and hyperostosis (BEIGHTON et al., 1976). Facial palsy may be a presenting feature in infancy and a patchy vertebral sclerosis is demonstrable in the neonate. Bony changes are not marked in the early stages but massive hyperostosis ultimately develops and the long term prognosis is poor.

References

BEIGHTON, P., CREMIN, B. J., HAMERSMA, H.: The radiology of sclerosteosis. Br. J. Radiol. **49**, 934 (1976).
BEIGHTON, P., HORAN, F. T., HAMERSMA, H.: The osteopetroses—a review. Postgrad. Med. J. **53**, 507 (1977).
CREMIN, B. J., FISHER, R. M.: The lesions of congenital syphilis. Br. J. Radiol. **43**, 333 (1970).
GOLBUS, M. S., KOERPER, M. A., HALL, B. D.: Failure to diagnosis osteopetrosis in utero. Lancet **1976/II**, 1246.
GRAHAM, C. B., RUDHE, U., EKLÜF, O.: Intrinsic diseases of bones. Progress in Pediatric Radiology. Osteopetrosis, Vol. IV, p. 375. Basel: Karger 1973.
JENKINSON, E. L., PFISTERER, W. H., LATTEIER, K. K., MARTIN, M.: A prenatal diagnosis of osteopetrosis. Am. J. Roentgenol. **49**, 455 (1943).
LORIA CORTES, R., QUESADA-CALVO, E., CORDERO-CHAVEM, C.: Osteopetrosis in children. A report of 26 cases. Pediatrics **91**, 43 (1977).
MAROTEAUX, P., LAMY, M.: La pycnodysostose. Presse Méd. **70**, 999 (1962).
NEUMAN, N., PIERSON, M., MARCHAL, C., MICHAUD, C.: Evolution and prognostic de la forme precose et grave de la maladie d'Albers Schönberg. Pediatrie **14**, 293 (1964).
SLY, W. S., LANG, R., ALVIOLI, L., HADDAD, J., LUBOWITZ, H., MCALISTER, W.: Recessive osteopetrosis: a new clinical phenotype. Am. J. Hum. Genet. **24**, 34 (1972).

Chapter 19 (Figs. 19-1a, b)

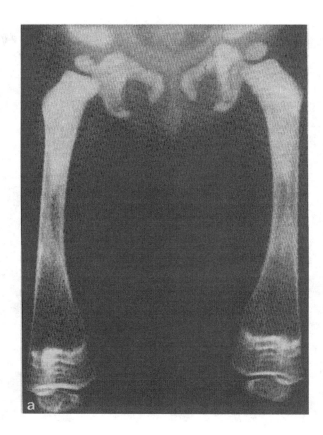

Case I

Fig. 19-1. (a) One-year-old infant. Sclerosis is evident in the pubis and upper femora. The lower femora show abnormal modeling and dense stratification

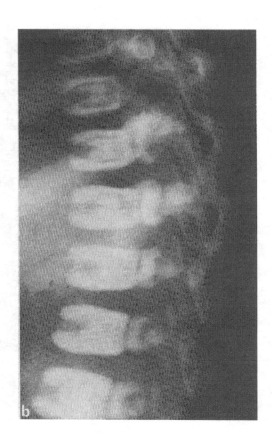

Fig. 19-1. (b) Vertebrae showing marked endo-bone formation with sclerosis of end plates

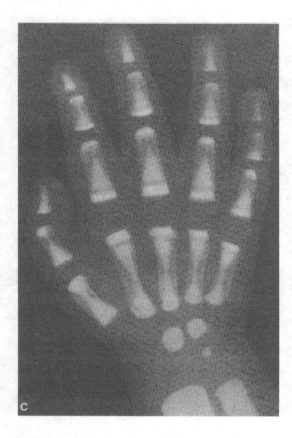

Case I

Fig. 19-1. (c) Hand showing metaphyseal sclerosis and endobone formation

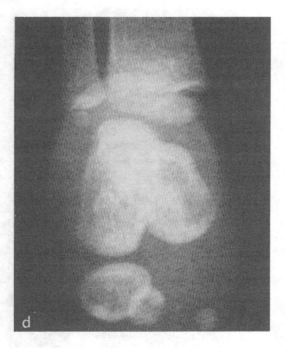

Fig. 19-1. (d) Ankle showing sclerotic margins to the round bones

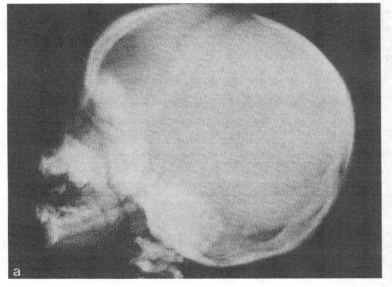
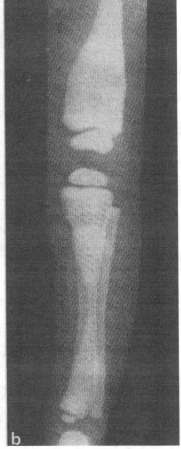

Case II

Fig. 19-2. (a) Two-year-old child with generalized sclerosis of the skull, maximal at the base. (b) Generalized sclerosis and abnormal modelling in the femur and tibia

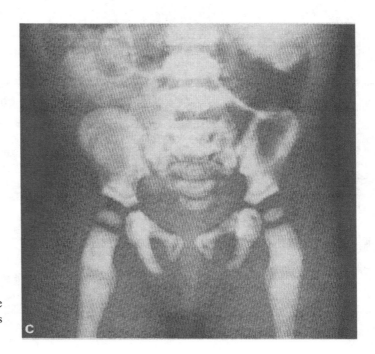

Fig. 19-2. (c) Pelvis with endobone formation in the ilia wings and sclerosis in the pubis and femora

Chapter 19 (Figs. 19-3a, b)

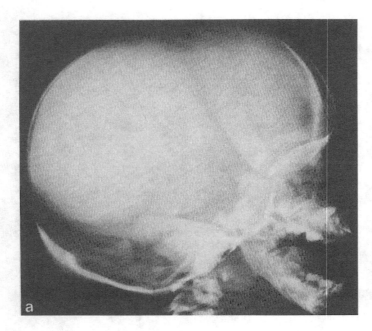

Case III

Fig. 19-3. (a) Pycnodysostosis. Skull of 1-year-old infant showing increased density with widely open sutures and anterior fontanelle. Angle of the mandible is typically flattened

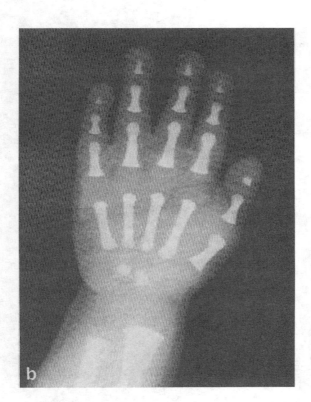

Fig. 19-3. (b) Hand showing generalized sclerosis, with growth failure of the terminal phalanges. Lack of modelling is not a feature of this condition

Chapter 19 (Fig. 19-4)

Case IV

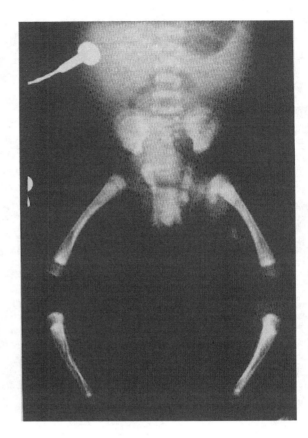

Fig. 19-4. Serologically proven case of congenital syphilis. Lucent areas in the metaphyses and iliac bones are nonspecific features of growth disturbance (dystrophy) and should not be confused with the stratification of osteopetrosis

Appendix

Monographs

BAILEY, JOSEPH, A. II.: Disproportionate Short Stature. Philadelphia-London-Toronto: W. B. Saunders Company 1973.
BEIGHTON, PETER: Inherited Disorders of the Skeleton. Edinburgh: Churchill Livingstone Company 1978.
BERGSMA, D. (Ed.): Skeletal Dysplasias, Vol. X, Nos 9 and 12. The National Foundation March of Dimes: New York 1974.
CARTER, C. O., FAIRBANK, T. J.: The Genetics of Locomotor Disorders. London-New York-Toronto: Oxford University Press 1974.
KAUFMAN, H. J. (Ed.): Progress in Pediatric Radiology, Intrinsic Diseases of Bones, Vol. IV. Basel-München-Paris-New York-Sydney: S. Karger 1973.
MAROTEAUX, PIERRE: Maldies Osseuses de L'Enfant. Paris: Flammarion Médicine-Sciences 1974.
McKUSICK, VICTOR A.: Heritable Disorders of Connective Tissue, 4th Ed. St. Louis: The C. V. Mosby Company 1972.
McKUSICK, VICTOR A.: Mendelian Inheritance in Man, 4th Ed. Baltimore-London: The Johns Hopkins Press 1975.
SMITH, DAVID W.: Recognisable Patterns of Human Malformation, 2nd Ed. Philadelphia-London-Toronto: W. B. Saunders Company 1976.
SPRANGER, JÜRGEN W., LANGER, LEONARD O., WIEDEMANN, H.-R.: Bone Dysplasias. Stuttgart: Gustav Fisher Verlag 1974.
WYNNE-DAVIES, RUTH., FAIRBANK, T. J.: Fairbank's Atlas of General Affections of the Skeleton, 2nd Ed. Edinburgh-London-New York: Churchill Livingstone 1976.

Reviews

CREMIN, B. J., BEIGHTON, P.: Dwarfism in the newborn: the nomenclature, radiological features and genetic significance. Br. J. Radiol. 47, 77 (1974).
CURRAN, J. P., SIGMON, B. A., OPITZ, J. M.: Lethal forms of chondrodysplastic dwarfism. Pediatr. 53/1, 76 (1974).
FELSON, BENJAMIN (Ed.): Seminars in Roentgenology. Dwarfs and Other Little People, 1973, Vol. VIII, No. 2.
HOUSTON, C. S., AWEN, C. F., KENT, H. P.: Fatal neonatal dwarfism. J. Can. Assoc. Radiol. 23, 45 (1972).
MAROTEAUX, P., STANESCU, V., STANESCU, R.: The lethal chondrodysplasias. Clin. Orthop. 114, 31 (1976).
MARTIN, C.: Osteochondrodysplasias recognisable at birth. Med. Infantile 82/1, 5 (1975).
YANG, S.-S., HEIDELBERGER, K. P., BROUGH, A. J., CORBETT, D. P., BERNSTEIN, J.: Perspective in Pediatric Pathology. Lethal Short-Limbed Chondrodysplasia in Early Infancy. In: ROSENBERG, H. S., BOLANDE, R. P. (Eds.): Year Book Medical Publishers, Chicago 1976, Vol. III.

Subject Index

Achondrogenesis   17, 18
Achondroplasia   55–60
   homozygous achondroplasia   56
Acromesomelic dysplasia   73
Albers-Schönberg disease 101
Amniocentesis   5
Amniography   10
Asphyxiating thoracic dysplasia
(Jeune syndrome)   27–31

Campomelic dysplasia   53–55
Chondroectodermal dysplasia
   (Ellis-van Creveld syndrome)   33–36
Chondrodysplasia punctata   45–51
   rhizomelic type   45
      Conradi-Hünermann type   46
   other types   47
Cleido-cranial dysplasia   83–89
Cloverleaf skull   22
Conradi-Hünermann type of
   chondrodysplasia punctata   46

Diastrophic dysplasia   61–65

Fetography   10
Fetoscopy   5

Grebe syndrome   17

Hypophosphatasia   97–99

Jeune syndrome (asphyxiating thoracic
   dysplasia)   27–31

Kleeblattschädel   22
Kniest syndrome   68

Larsen syndrome   79–81

Mesomelic dysplasia   73–77
   acrodysplasia   74
   acromesomelic dysplasia   73
   peripheral dysostosis   73
Metatropic dysplasia   67–70
   Kniest syndrome   68
   pseudometatropic dysplasia   67
      Weissenbacher-Zweymuller
      syndrome   68
Morquio syndrome   71

Osteogenesis imperfecta congenita   91–95
Osteopetrosis   101–107

Peripheral dysostosis   73
Pseudometatropic dysplasia   67
Pycnodysostosis   101

Sclerosteosis   101
Short rib-polydactyly syndromes   37–44
   Saldino-Noonan, Majewski, and
   Naumoff types   37
Spondyleopiphyseal dysplasia congenita
   71–73

Thanatophoric dysplasia   21–26

Ultrasonography   10

Current Diagnostic Pediatrics

Series Editor: A. Chrispin

Volume 1

Current Concepts in Pediatric Radiology

Editor: O. Eklöf

With contributions by R. Astley, V. Boston, D. Brockwell, S. Candranel, A. R. Chrispin, M. Cremer, N. Cremer, B. J. Cremin, C. Fauré, H. Fendel, A. Giedion, B. R. Girdany, G. B. C. Harris, M. Hassan, M. A. Lassrich, W. Porstmann, A. K. Poznanski, P. Rodesch, F. N. Silverman, G. Theander

1977. 165 figures in 265 separate illustrations, 12 tables.
X, 150 pages
ISBN 3-540-08279-4

Contents: Radiology of Respiratory Distress in the Newborn. – A "Gamut of Pattern" Approach. – Chronic Lung Disorders in II. Childhood. – Therapeutic Embolization of Arteriovenous Pulmonary Fistolas by Catheter Technique. – Pediatric Gastrointestinal Fiberendoscopy. – The Esophagus in Infancy. – Less Common Disease Patterns in the Gastro-Intestinal Tract with a Special Note on Meconium Ileus. – Small Intestine – The Terminal Ileum Loop. – Current Views on the Diagnosis of Colonic Aganglionosis. – Renal Cysts and Cystlike Conditions in Infancy and Childhood. – Aspects of Acute Kidney Injury in Young Infants. – The Radiology of the Vesico-Ureteric Junction. – The Prostate in Pediatric Radiology. – Approaches to the Evaluation of the Hand in the Congenital Malformation Syndromes. – Lesions of the Spine. – A Radiological Study. – Hydrocephalus in Children.

All who wish to know what is important and current in pediatric radiology will need to have this volume. Dr. Eklöf of the Karolinska Hospital, Stockholm, has assembled an international team of outstanding contributors. They write on a wide variety of subjects and define the frontiers reached by recent advances. *Current Concepts in Pediatric Radiology* shows that radiology has a cardinal role in almost every investigation and evaluation of childhood disease. The knowledge in this book is of interest and concern to each radiologist, pediatrician, and pediatric surgeon who needs an account of what is contemporary and important. *Current Concepts in Pediatric Radiology* marks the start of a new series by Springer International. The objective of the series *Current Diagnostic Pediatrics,* is to communicate knowledge of investigation and evaluation in the wide range of disease in children.

Current Concepts in Pediatric Radiology is the No. 1 volume in the new Springer International series *Current Diagnostic Pediatrics.* Subsequent volumes in preparation include *Gastroenterology, Trauma, Urology* and *Heart Disease.*

Springer International

Handbuch der medizinischen Radiologie

Encyclopedia of Medical Radiology

Herausgeber: L. Diethelm, F. Heuck, O. Olsson, K. Ranniger, F. Strnad, H. Vieten, A. Zuppinger

Band 5

Röntgendiagnostik der Skeleterkrankungen
Diseases of the Skeletal System (Roentgen Diagnosis)

Teil 6

Bone Tumors

By M.C. Beachley, M.H. Becker, P.A. Collins, K. Doi, H.F. Faunce, F. Feldman, H. Firooznia, E.W. Fordham, H.K. Genant, N.B. Genieser, A. Goldman, G.B. Greenfield, H.J. Griffiths, J.P. Petasnick, P.J. Pevsner, R.S. Pinto, P.C. Ramachandran, F. Schajowicz, I. Yaghmai

Edited by K. Ranniger

1977. 639 figures (1086 separate illustrations).
XXI, 825 pages
ISBN 3-540-08312-X

In this volume, 20 prominent radiologists discuss benign and malignant bone tumors with respect to pathological anatomy, morphology, and histology. The editing of the difficult and often contradictory information has focused on the differing viewpoints held by radiologists and pathologists as to the cause of, varying terminology for, and classification of tumors. In each chapter the authors evaluate the results of research in these fields to establish criteria for an absolute diagnosis. The difficulties in differential diagnosis and the development of individual bone tumors (as observed radiologically in various stages) are discussed at length. Each chapter is clearly arranged and illustrated with excellent figures, skillful drawings, and easy-to-read tables. This handbook volume will thus be extremely valuable, not only to specialties involved with morphology such as radiology such as radiology and pathology, but to all medical disciplines generally concerned with the diagnosis and treatment of tumors.

New Concepts in Maxillofacial Bone Surgery

From the Unit of Maxillofacial Surgery, Division of Plastic and Reconstructive Surgery, Department of Surgery of the University of Basle

Edited by B. Spiessl

Contributors:
C. Bassetti, Basle – D. Cornoley, Berne –
T. Gensheimer, Basle – H. Graf, Berne –
E. Holtgrave, Bonn – W. Huser, Olten –
W.-A. Jaques, Basle – G. Martinoni, Basle –
R. Mathys, Bettlach – J. Prein, Basle – T. Rakosi, Freiburg – W. Remagen, Basle – R. Schmoker, Basle – B. Spiessl, Basle – H.M. Tschopp, Basle

1976. 183 figures, 36 tables. XIII, 194 pages
ISBN 3-540-07929-7

The present volume is concerned with bone surgery in the area of the facial skeleton. The focus is on the search for practical solutions to the problem of stability.

The main idea is to recognize that primary consolidation of fragments in fractures or osteotomies, as well as undisturbed revascularization of bone transplants and long-term tolerance of inert implants or joint prostheses, *depend on the stability of fixation.*

The clinical questions which follow are presented in individual contributions in the form of firm principles, selected cases, or experimental studies.

Of particular value are the detailed illustrations of the operative steps. In this connection newly developed sets of instruments are illustrated whose use facilitates an exact procedure.

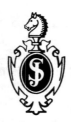

Springer-Verlag
Berlin Heidelberg New York

Printed by Publishers' Graphics LLC